FIBROMYALGIA

The Cause & The Cure

Annesse Brockley
and
Kristin Urdiales

Nature Had It First

FIBROMYALGIA
THE CAUSE AND THE CURE
By Annesse Brockley and Kristin Urdiales

Printed in the United States of America

First Edition
10 9 8 7 6 5 4 3 2 1

Website: www.NatureHadItFirst.com

Published by Nature Had It First
195 Pine Cone Ave
Spearfish, SD 57783
ISBN: 978-0-9836037-5-7

Message to the Reader

Neither the publisher, nor the authors are engaged in rendering professional advice or services to the reader. This book is not intended as a substitute for medical advice from a licensed health care practitioner. Any decision involving the treatment of an illness should be made only after consulting a physician. Do not adjust your medication in any way without professional medical advice. The reader should consult his or her medical, health, or other competent professional before adopting any of the suggestions in this book or drawing inferences from it. The authors and publisher specifically disclaim all responsibility for any liability, loss, or risk, personal or otherwise, which is incurred as a consequence, directly or indirectly, of the use and application of any of the contents of this book.

Dedication and Acknowledgements

This book is dedicated to the many sufferers of fibromyalgia.

To our family and friends –thank you for your love and support.

Above all, we thank The God of All Comfort.

From the Authors

This book has brought together scientific research from around the world, which we believe uncovers the cause of fibromyalgia. Every symptom of fibromyalgia can now be clearly explained and traced back to its origin. This collective evidence offers valid proof, not only of the cause of fibromyalgia, but also of the only possible way to cure it.

— Annesse Brockley and Kristin Urdiales

Contents

Section One: The Cause

Section Two: The Cure

Guide to Recipes

SECTION 1

THE CAUSE

CHAPTER 1

Fibromyalgia: The Cause

If you've been diagnosed with fibromyalgia, I know how sick you are. When I first became sick over twenty years ago, my initial diagnosis was fibromyalgia and chronic fatigue syndrome. After a few years I developed a malar rash, which then led to an additional diagnosis of lupus.

I think it is fair to say that many people don't consider fibromyalgia a "serious" illness. Others may think that your illness is primarily psychosomatic.

As a patient with fibromyalgia, I was interviewed once by a doctor on a radio show that began my interview by saying to millions of people, "I am not calling you crazy, but..." She then focused her entire line of questioning to me on the basis that I must have been abused as a child. I wasn't.

The information in this book should set the record straight on whether or not fibromyalgia is a "real" disease. It is not only real, it is many of the things you have been told it is not. It is progressive and inflammatory. It is linked to heart disease and cancer.

I had a burning desire to know "why" I was sick. My prayers were answered. I know why and I want you to know why too. Every symptom of fibromyalgia will be clearly and completely explained. The numerous valid scientific findings in fibromyalgia will lead the way. We will be able to show that each finding can be traced directly back to one source. That source is missing digestive enzymes called protease.

We will begin by listing the valid scientific findings in fibromyalgia. We will be providing studies as evidence of these findings. In turn, these findings will lead to the many symptoms found in fibromyalgia.

FIBROMYALGIA SCIENTIFIC FINDINGS

- Lack of essential amino acids
- Low serotonin
- Low melatonin
- Low dopamine
- Low adrenal function
- Brain grey matter loss
- Hypothyroidism
- Mitochrondrial dysfunction
- Low ATP
- Reduced CoQ10
- Low carnitine
- Low glutathione
- Low serum ferritin
- Low muscle oxygenation
- Restless legs syndrome
- Spinal cord degeneration
- Carpal tunnel syndrome
- Low vitamin B12
- Autonomic nervous system dysfunction (dysautonomia)
- Postural orthostatic tachycardia syndrome (POTS)
- Overactive bladder
- Dry eyes and mouth
- Sleep apnea
- Migraines and headaches
- Elevated substance P
- Raynaud's phenomenon
- Low intracellular magnesium
- Elevated homocysteine
- Decreased levels of collagen cross-linking
- Temporomandibular joint disorder (TMJ)

- Mitral valve prolapse
- Hypermobility
- Excess nitric oxide
- Endometriosis
- Increased risk of cancer
- Elevated tumor necrosis factor (TNF)
- Allodynia
- Excessive daytime sleepiness
- Chronic urticaria (hives)
- Allergies
- Inflammatory bowel disease
- Low GABA
- Anxiety
- Association with ADHD
- Sound sensitivity
- Severe premenstrual syndrome
- Elevated glutamate
- Depression
- Bipolar disorder
- Increased risk of suicide
- Irritable bowel syndrome
- Interstitial cystitis
- Inflammation of the fascia
- Increased kynurenine pathway activity
- Low growth hormone secretion
- Low somatomedin C
- Low endorphins
- Comorbidity with rheumatoid arthritis
- Osteoporosis
- Low calcium
- Low vitamin D
- Low zinc
- Low stomach acid
- Small intestine bacterial overgrowth (SIBO)
- Increased intestinal permeability
- Multiple chemical sensitivity
- Low cortisol
- Low estrogen
- Low DHEA
- Low testosterone
- Comorbidity with lupus
- Abnormal proteins

LACK OF ESSENTIAL AMINO ACIDS

Our first scientific finding is *lack of essential amino acids*. An essential amino acid is an amino acid that cannot be synthesized by the body and therefore must be supplied in the diet. Amino acids are the fundamental building blocks for every cell in the body. There are nine essential amino acids:

- Phenylalanine
- Tryptophan
- Methionine
- Leucine
- Isoleucine
- Valine
- Lysine
- Histidine
- Threonine

Essential amino acids are found in foods that contain proteins. Protease (digestive enzymes) digest dietary proteins and release essential amino acids. A lack of protease would therefore lead to a lack of essential amino acids.

Studies confirm that fibromyalgia (FM) patients lack numerous essential amino acids (AAs). In the following study entitled "Altered amino acid homeostasis in subjects affected by fibromyalgia" researchers found that fibromyalgia patients had significantly lower levels of the essential amino acids valine, methionine, phenylalanine, and threonine. The patients also lacked the amino acid tyrosine. Tyrosine is an amino acid the body makes from the essential amino acid phenylalanine.

STUDY

Altered amino acid homeostasis in subjects affected by fibromyalgia.

Bazzichi, L., L. Palego, G. Giannaccini, A. Rossi, F. De Feo, C. Giacomelli, L. Betti, L. Giusti, G. Mascia, S. Bombardieri, A. Lucacchini. 2009. *Clin Bioche.* 42(10-11):1064-70.

"Significant lower plasma...tyrosine (Tyr), valine, methionine, phenylalanine and threonine concentrations, and the sum of essential AAs were observed in FM patients vs. healthy controls..."

In our next study researchers found that patients with fibromyalgia lacked the essential amino acids phenylalanine, leucine, isoleucine, and valine. Leucine, isoleucine, and valine are the three branched chain amino acids (BCAAs). The term "branched chain" refers to their molecular structure. The BCAAs are used by the muscles for energy and in the regulation of protein synthesis.

STUDY

Serotonergic markers and lowered plasma branched-chain-amino acid concentrations in fibromyalgia.

Maes, M.R. Verkerk, L. Delmeire, A. Van Gastel, F. van Hunsel, S. Scharpé. 2000. *Psychiatry Res.* Dec 4;97(1):11-20.

"Patients with fibromyalgia had significantly lower plasma concentrations of the three BCAAs (valine, leucine and isoleucine) and phenylalanine than normal controls. It is hypothesized that the relative deficiency in the BCAAs may play a role in the pathophysiology of fibromyalgia, since the BCAAs supply energy to the muscle and regulate protein synthesis in the muscles."

Fibromyalgia patients also lack the essential amino acids tryptophan and histidine. In the following study published in the *Journal of Rheumatology* researchers found that fibromyalgia patients were deficient in tryptophan and histidine.

STUDY

Plasma tryptophan and other amino acids in primary fibromyalgia: a controlled study.

Yunus M.B., J.W. Dailey, J.C. Aldag, A.T. Masi, P.C. Jobe. 1992. *J Rheumatol* Jan;19(1):90-4.

"Transport ratio of tryptophan was found to be significantly...decreased in PF compared with the control group...Plasma tryptophan level was lower in PF... than in healthy controls... Additionally, plasma histidine... levels were found to be significantly...lower in patients with PF than in controls."

Our studies have shown that fibromyalgia patients are deficient in the following amino acids:

- Tryptophan
- Phenylalanine
- Tyrosine
- Leucine
- Isoleucine
- Valine
- Methionine
- Threonine
- Histidine

These missing amino acids would account for many of the other scientific findings and symptoms found in fibromyalgia. For instance, as Figure 1 demonstrates, the essential amino acid tryptophan is needed to produce *serotonin*, which is our next scientific finding.

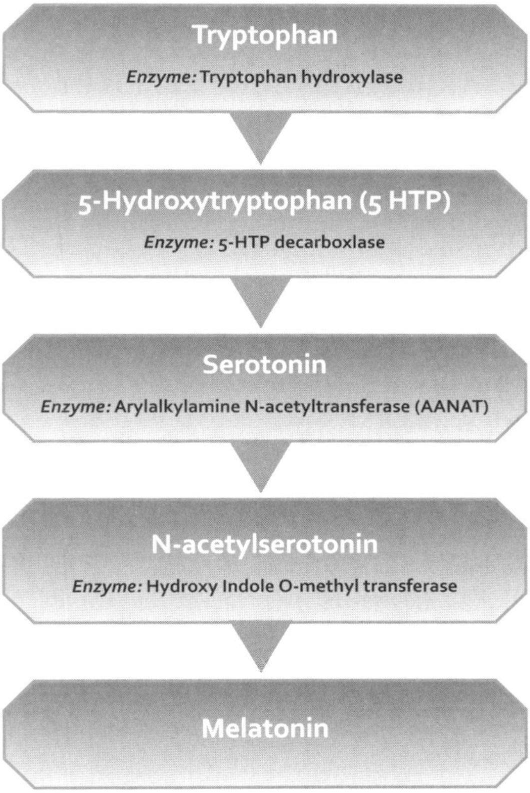

Figure 1. Demonstrated here is the production of serotonin and melatonin from the amino acid tryptophan.

Low Serotonin

The following study confirms that fibromyalgia (FM) patients have significantly lower levels of serotonin.

STUDY

Serotonin levels, pain threshold, and fibromyalgia symptoms in the general population.

Wolfe, F., I.J. Russell, G. Vipraio, K. Ross, J. Anderson. 1997. *J Rheumatol* 24(3):555-9.

"Serum serotonin levels are significantly lower in persons with FM compared to those without FM..."

The lack of serotonin would then account for some of the symptoms found in fibromyalgia.

SYMPTOMS OF LOW SEROTONIN

- Inability to fall and stay asleep
- Excessive worrying
- Cognitive impairment (inability to focus, poor memory, lack of mental clarity)
- Anxiety in typically low stress situations
- Fatigue in spite of adequate rest
- Mood swings
- Irritability
- Moderate to overwhelming sadness

LOW MELATONIN

Tryptophan and serotonin are also needed to produce the hormone *melatonin* (see Figure 1), which is an important factor in a good night's rest.

The following study found that fibromyalgia syndrome (FMS) patients had a 31% lower nocturnal melatonin (MT) secretion than healthy subjects.

STUDY

Fibromyalgia—a syndrome associated with decreased nocturnal melatonin secretion.

Wikner, J., U. Hirsch, L. Wetterberg, S. Röjdmark. 1998. *Clin Endocrinol (Oxf)* 49(2):179-83.

> "The FMS patients had a 31% lower MT secretion than healthy subjects during the hours of darkness."

SYMPTOMS OF LOW MELATONIN
• Insomnia • Difficulty getting to sleep • Difficulty falling back to sleep when awakened during the night • Light sleeper/easy waking during the night • Early morning awakening • Un-refreshing sleep • Lack of dreaming

Low Dopamine

The essential amino acid phenylalanine is needed to produce *dopamine*—our next scientific finding.

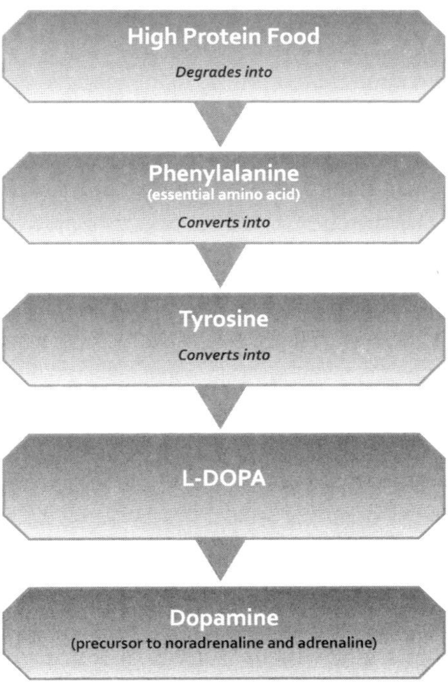

Figure 2.
Diagram illustrating the relationship between dopamine synthesis and dietary proteins.

In the following study published in *The Journal of Pain*, Dr. Patrick Wood, a former scientific advisor for the National Fibromyalgia Association, found that the brains of people with fibromyalgia syndrome (FMS) have reduced levels of dopamine.

STUDY

Reduced presynaptic dopamine activity in fibromyalgia syndrome demonstrated with positron emission tomography: a pilot study.

Wood, P.B., J.C. Patterson 2nd, J.J. Sunderland, K.H. Tainter, M.F. Glabus, D.L. Lilien. 2007. *J Pain* 8(1):51-8. Epub 2006 Oct 4.

"It appears that FMS might be characterized by a disruption of dopaminergic neurotransmission...An association between FMS and reduced dopamine metabolism within the pain neuromatrix provides important insights into the pathophysiology of this mysterious disorder."

SYMPTOMS OF LOW DOPAMINE

- Stiff, rigid, achy muscles
- Cognitive impairment
- Impaired motor skills
- Tremors
- Inability to focus attention
- Poor balance and coordination
- Strange walking pattern (gait), frequently with small steps

Low Adrenal Function

The lack of dopamine would explain the *low adrenal function* often found in patients with fibromyalgia (Wingenfeld, 2008). Dopamine is the precursor to both of the adrenal hormones-adrenaline and noradrenaline (see Figure 2).

SYMPTOMS OF LOW ADRENALINE AND NORADRENALINE	
• Fatigue	• Weakness
• Lack of concentration and motivation	• Nausea
• Problems with losing weight	• Dizziness
• Depression	• Salt cravings

Brain Gray Matter Loss

Low dopamine is also associated with *brain gray matter loss,* our next scientific finding. The gray matter involves regions of the brain concerned with muscle control, emotions, learning and memory, speech, and sensory perception, such as seeing and hearing.

In the following study published in the *Journal of Neuroscience* researchers found that the longer the individuals had fibromyalgia, the greater the brain gray matter loss, with each year of fibromyalgia being equivalent to 9.5 times the loss in normal aging.

STUDY

Accelerated brain gray matter loss in fibromyalgia patients: premature aging of the brain?

Kuchinad, A. P. Schweinhardt, D.A. Seminowicz, P.B. Wood, B.A. Chizh, M.C. Bushnell. 2007. *J Neurosci* 11;27(15):4004-7.

"We found that fibromyalgia patients had significantly less total gray matter volume and showed a 3.3 times greater age-associated decrease in gray matter than healthy controls. The longer the individuals had had fibromyalgia, the greater the gray matter loss, with each year of fibromyalgia being equivalent to 9.5 times the loss in normal aging."

In our next study, published in the *Journal of Pain,* researchers found a strong correlation between dopamine metabolism and gray matter density.

STUDY

Changes in gray matter density in fibromyalgia: correlation with dopamine metabolism.

Wood, P.B., M.F. Glabus, R. Simpson, J.C. Patterson 2nd. 2009. *J Pain* 10(6):609-18. Epub 2009 Apr 23.

"Fibromyalgia is associated with reductions in gray matter density within brain regions ostensibly involved in phenomena related to the disorder, including enhanced pain perception, cognitive dysfunction, and abnormal stress reactivity. Given mounting evidence of abnormal dopaminergic neurotransmission associated with the disorder, the strong correlation between dopamine metabolism and gray matter density provides insight as to the pathophysiology that might contribute to these changes."

HYPOTHYROIDISM

The lack of the essential amino acid phenylalanine would also explain the association fibromyalgia has with our next scientific finding—*hypothyroidism*. According to the National Institutes of Health, hypothyroidism is an associated disorder of fibromyalgia (Bazzichi, 2012).

Phenylalanine is not only needed for the synthesis of dopamine and both of the adrenal hormones, it is also required for the synthesis of both of the thyroid hormones. Phenylalanine is converted into tyrosine and tyrosine is then used for the synthesis of the thyroid hormones—thyroxine and triiodothyronine.

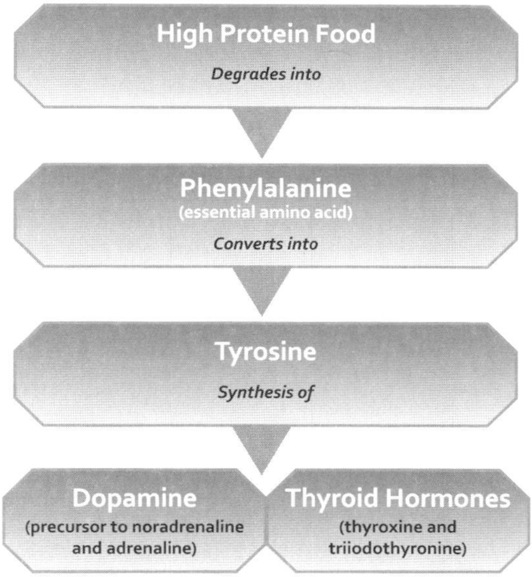

Figure 3.
Diagram demonstrating the production of the thyroid hormones from the amino acid tyrosine.

SYMPTOMS OF HYPOTHYROIDISM

- Sensitivity to cold
- Constipation
- Depression
- Fatigue
- Dry, pale skin
- Thin, brittle hair and fingernails
- Weight gain
- Joint or muscle pain
- Heavier menstrual periods

As our studies have shown, fibromyalgia patients lack numerous essential amino acids. These essential amino acids are derived from dietary proteins. Protease are responsible for the digestion of dietary proteins and subsequent release of essential amino acids. These essential amino acids are needed to supply energy to the muscles and for the production of important hormones and neurotransmitters, such as dopamine, serotonin, melatonin, and both the thyroid and the adrenal hormones. The lack of these essential amino acids, hormones, and neurotransmitters would then lead to many of the symptoms found in fibromyalgia, such as muscle weakness and fatigue, insomnia, anxiety, joint and muscle pain, poor balance and coordination, nausea, irritability, fatigue etc.

CHAPTER 2

Scientific Findings:

Mitochondrial Dysfunction, Low ATP, Reduced CoQ10, Low Carnitine, and Low Glutathione

---

OUR NEXT SCIENTIFIC FINDINGS ARE mitochrondrial dysfunction, low ATP, reduced CoQ10, low carnitine, and low glutathione.

MITOCHONDRIAL DYSFUNCTION

The inability to produce either the thyroid or the adrenal hormones would partly explain one of the most devastating symptoms of fibromyalgia-fatigue. Someone who lives with fibromyalgia, though, knows that the fatigue is at the deepest levels of the cells. This type of fatigue would be explained by *mitochrondrial dysfunction*.

Mitochondria are structures that are found inside virtually every cell in the body. They lie at the very center of the body's ability to create energy. The researchers state in the following study, "In most cases, mitochondrial morphologic alterations have been found in muscle biopsies from FM patients."

STUDY

The role of oxidative stress and mitochondrial dysfunction in the pathogenesis of fibromyalgia.

Cordero, M.D., M.D. Miguel, I. Carmona-López, P. Bonal, F. Campa, A.M. Moreno-Fernández. 2010. *Neuro Endocrinlogy Letters* 31(2):169-173.

"In most cases, mitochondrial morphologic alterations have been found in muscle biopsies from FM patients."

Low ATP

Essential amino acids are needed to produce critical compounds for the mitochrondria, such as Coenzyme Q10 (CoQ10), carnitine, and glutathione. Without these compounds the mitochrondria would not be able to produce *adenosine triphosphate (ATP),* which is the currency of energy in the body. The following study from Vanderbilt University found significantly lower levels of ATP in the muscles of patients with fibromyalgia.

STUDY

Use of P-31 magnetic resonance spectroscopy to detect metabolic abnormalities in muscles of patients with fibromyalgia.

Park, J.H., P. Phothimat, C.T. Oates, M. Hernanz-Schulman, N.J. Olsen. 1998. *Arthritis Rheum* 41(3):406-13.

"patients had significantly lower than normal...ATP levels...in the quadriceps muscles during rest."

Significantly lower ATP levels have also been found in the platelets of fibromyalgia patients. The following study found that platelet ATP levels were 80% higher in healthy controls than in fibromyalgia patients.

STUDY

ATP, calcium and magnesium levels in platelets of patients with primary fibromyalgia.

Bazzichi, L., G. Giannaccini, L. Betti, L. Fabbrini, L. Schmid, L. Palego, C. Giacomelli, A. Rossi, L. Giusti, F. De Feo, T. Giuliano, G. Mascia, S. Bombardieri, A. Lucacchini. 2008. *Clin Biochem* 41(13):1084-90. Epub 2008 Jul 2.

"Significantly lower ATP levels were observed inside platelets of FM patients..."

Reduced CoQ10

Coenzyme Q10 is one of the essential nutrients needed by the mitochondria to produce ATP. Coenzyme Q10 acts as an essential cofactor in the production of ATP. In addition, it is an important antioxidant that protects the mitochondria from oxidative damage (Quinzii, 2010).

In the following study researchers found reduced levels of coenzyme Q10 and decreased mitochondrial membrane potential in fibromyalgia patients. Mitochondrial membrane potential is a key indicator of the cell's health.

STUDY

Mitochondrial dysfunction and mitophagy activation in blood mononuclear cells of fibromyalgia patients: implications in the pathogenesis of the disease.

Cordero, M.D., M. De Miguel, A.M. Moreno Fernández, I.M. Carmona López, J.G. Maraver, D. Cotán, L.G. Izquierdo, P. Bonal, Francisco Campa, P. Bullon, P. Navas, J.A. Sánchez Alcázar. 2010. *Arthritis Res Ther* 12(1): R17. Published online 2010 January 28.

"We found reduced levels of coenzyme Q10, decreased mitochondrial membrane potential..."

Coenzyme Q10 (CoQ10) is a fat-soluble compound synthesized by the body and also consumed in the diet. A report from Iowa State University lists beef, chicken, pork, and fish as the foods with the highest levels of CoQ10. Protease would be necessary to release CoQ10 from these high protein foods.

Coenzyme Q10 can also be synthesized by the body, but it requires the presence of one of two amino acids we have found lacking in fibromyalgia-phenylalanine or tyrosine.

According to the Linus Pauling Institute's Micronutrient Information Center at Oregon State University, one of the major steps involved in the biosynthesis of CoQ10 requires either phenylalanine or tyrosine (Higdon, 2003).

Tyrosine is derived from phenylalanine, and phenylalanine is found in high protein foods. Without the ability to break down high protein foods, you would not have the necessary amino acids to produce CoQ10.

Low Carnitine

Another critical compound necessary for the proper functioning of the mitochondria is *carnitine*. It is used by the mitochondria to produce ATP and in the export of toxic waste materials from the cell. The body manufactures carnitine from the essential amino acids lysine and methionine. We have shown that fibromyalgia patients lack the essential amino acid methionine.

Low levels of the carnitine compound, acylcarnitine, in the blood or muscles of people with CFS/FMS, have been found in the following studies:

1. Plioplys, A.V., S. Plioplys. 1997. Amantadine and L-Carnitine Treatment of Chronic Fatigue Syndrome. *Neuropsychobiology* 35(1):16-23.

2. Kuratsune, H., K. Yamaguti, M. Takahashi, et al. 1994. Acylcarnitine Deficiency in Chronic Fatigue Syndrome. *Clinical Infectious Disease* 18(3 Supplement 1): S62-S67.

3. Reuter, S.E., A.M. Evans. 2010. Long-chain Acylcarnitine Deficiency in Patients with Chronic Fatigue Syndrome. Potential Involvement of Altered Carnitine Palmitoyltransferase-I Activity. *Journal of Internal Medicine*:1365-2796

Low Glutathione

The essential amino acid methionine is also needed to produce *glutathione*. Glutathione is an antioxidant that helps the mitochondria avoid or repair damage that would normally lead to mitochondrial dysfunction and cell death. Methionine is a precursor for cysteine, and cysteine is a precursor for glutathione. In the following study glutathione levels were found to be "significantly" lower in fibromyalgia (FM) patients.

STUDY

Serum antioxidants and nitric oxide levels in fibromyalgia: a controlled study.

Sendur, O.F., Y. Turan, E. Tastaban, C. Yenisey, M. Serter. 2009. *Rheumatol Int.* 29(6):629-33. Epub 2008 Oct 14.

"Serum glutathione... levels were significantly lower in FM patients than controls. Additionally, the correlation between glutathione level and morning stiffness was found to be significant."

The lack of CoQ10, carnitine, and glutathione would clearly explain the mitochondrial dysfunction and low ATP found in fibromyalgia. Mitochondrial dysfunction would not only explain the profound fatigue associated with fibromyalgia, it would explain other symptoms found in fibromyalgia as well. Mitochondrial dysfunction would lead to such symptoms as exercise intolerance, muscle pain, cramping and weakness, feeling of extreme heaviness in the muscles, post-exertional malaise, hypotonia (loss of muscle tone), breathing difficulties, sensorineural hearing loss, and vision problems.

Mitochondrial dysfunction would also explain another devastating symptom of fibromyalgia-brain fog. All cells of the human body depend on ATP to provide energy. This is true for muscle cells, which provide movement, and nerve cells, which provide thought. Neurons, the brain cells that communicate with each other, have a high demand for energy because they are always in a state of metabolic activity. Even during sleep, neurons are still hard at work repairing and rebuilding their structural components. Altered energy metabolism would lead to mental confusion or lack of mental clarity. This is commonly known as "brain fog."

Patients with mitochondrial dysfunction might be able to muster some energy for periods of time, but it is generally short-lived and they tire quickly.

CHAPTER 3

Scientific Findings:
Low Serum Ferritin, Low Muscle Oxygenation, and Restless Legs Syndrome

---

OUR NEXT SCIENTIFIC FINDINGS ARE low serum ferritin, low muscle oxygenation, and restless legs syndrome.

LOW SERUM FERRITIN

The following study, published in the *European Journal of Clinical Nutrition*, found a significant difference in serum ferritin levels between healthy people and those with fibromyalgia. The researchers concluded that low ferritin created a 6.5 fold increase to the risk of fibromyalgia.

STUDY

Association between serum ferritin level and fibromyalgia syndrome.

Ortancil, O. A. Sanli, R. Eryuksel, A. Basaran, H. Ankarali. 2010. *Eur J Clin Nutr.* Mar;64(3):308-12. doi: 10.1038/ejcn.2009.149. Epub 2010 Jan 20.

> "The mean serum ferritin levels in the fibromyalgia (FM) and control groups were 27.3+/-20.9 and 43.8+/-30.8 ng/ml, respectively, and the difference was statistically significant (P=0.003)...having a serum ferritin level <50 ng/ml caused a 6.5-fold increased risk for FMS."

Ferritin is a protein in the body that binds to iron and serves to store iron in a nontoxic form. The amount of ferritin in the blood "normally" shows how much iron is stored in the body. This is true only if the body is properly metabolizing iron. The body will also "pull" ferritin from the bloodstream if it needs to protect cells from iron overload. According to Dr. Patrick Wood, a former scientific advisor for the National Fibromyalgia Association, a growing body of evidence suggests abnormal iron metabolism in fibromyalgia. In either case, *low serum ferritin* is an indicator of the body's access to bioavailable iron.

SYMPTOMS OF IRON DEFICIENCY

- Weakness and fatigue
- Shortness of breath
- Pruritus (itchiness)
- Rapid heartbeat
- Dizziness
- Cold hands and feet
- Severe menstrual pain and bleeding
- Hair loss
- Angina (chest pain)
- Inflamed or sore tongue

Low Muscle Oxygenation

A molecule of iron is needed to make an essential component of red blood cells called hemoglobin. Hemoglobin is a protein that carries oxygen in the red blood cell. The ability to exercise and even to generate energy for normal activity depends on adequate delivery of oxygen to cells. The following study confirms that fibromyalgia patients have *low muscle oxygenation*.

STUDY

Muscle tissue oxygen pressure in primary fibromyalgia.

Lund, N. A. Bengtsson, P. Thorborg. 1986. *Scand J Rheumatol* 15(2):165-73.

"The conclusion is that in patients with primary fibromyalgia, the muscle oxygenation is abnormal or low..."

Restless Legs Syndrome

The lack of iron and dopamine would lead to a condition commonly found in fibromyalgia-*restless legs syndrome*. A study published in the *Journal of Sleep Medicine* found that 33% of people with fibromyalgia also had restless legs syndrome (Viola-Saltzman, 2010).

In the following study from Johns Hopkins entitled "Dopamine and iron in the pathophysiology of restless legs syndrome (RLS)" the researchers state, "It is concluded that there may be an iron-dopamine connection central to the pathophysiology of RLS for at least some if not most patients with this disorder."

STUDY

Dopamine and iron in the pathophysiology of restless legs syndrome (RLS).

Allen, R. 2004. *Sleep Med.* 5(4):385-91.

"It is concluded that there may be an iron-dopamine connection central to the pathophysiology of RLS for at least some if not most patients with this disorder."

In addition to breaking down proteins and releasing essential amino acids, protease are also responsible for regulating iron absorption in the body. Without these enzymes, the body would not be able to properly metabolize iron. The following study entitled "New insights into intestinal iron absorption" concludes that protease are an essential component of a pathway that detects iron deficiency and regulates iron absorption in the body. The inability to properly metabolize iron led to the mouse in the study developing not only anemia, but also a progressive loss of body hair. Iron is the single nutrient most often associated with hair loss, a common symptom of fibromyalgia, since it is necessary for the production of proteins that make up a strand of hair.

STUDY

New insights into intestinal iron absorption.

Hörl, W.H. 2008. *Nephrol. Dial. Transplant.* 23(10):3063-3064.

"Take home message: Iron deficiency activates the serine protease TMPRSS6. The protease then inhibits hepcidin transcription and thereby allows intestinal iron absorption and cellular iron release."

As the study confirms, protease are essential for iron absorption and cellular iron release. The lack of protease would lead not only to a lack of bioavailable iron, it would also lead to iron overload within the cells. Unbound iron is toxic to the cells, so the body will pull the binding protein, ferritin, from the blood into the cells in an attempt to prevent cell damage. This would lead to low serum levels of ferritin, but would not be indicative of the amount of iron in the cells.

Numerous studies have shown that cellular iron overload plays a major role in stimulating cancer. In the study entitled "The role of iron in cancer" the researchers state, "The metal is carcinogenic due to its catalytic effect on the formation of hydroxyl radicals, suppression of the activity of host defense cells and promotion of cancer cell multiplication. In both animals and humans, primary neoplasms develop at body sites of excessive iron deposits" (Weinburg, 1996).

A low serum level of iron in fibromyalgia may very well be due to toxic overload within the cells, so we wouldn't want to ingest more iron in supplement form in an attempt to restore blood iron levels.

CHAPTER 4

Scientific Findings:

Spinal Cord Degeneration, Carpal Tunnel Syndrome, and Low Vitamin B12

OUR NEXT SCIENTIFIC FINDINGS ARE spinal cord degeneration, carpal tunnel syndrome, and low vitamin B12.

SPINAL CORD DEGENERATION

Spinal cord degeneration is another one of Dr. Wood's (former scientific advisor for the National Fibromyalgia Association) findings. We spoke with him and asked if he was referring to subacute combined degeneration of the spinal cord. He stated he was. The reason why the disease is "combined" is because both sensory and motor nerves are affected. Numbness, tingling, and a burning pain of the extremities are common symptoms of sensory nerve involvement. Muscle weakness, muscle stiffness, cramps and spasms are common symptoms of motor nerve involvement.

Damage to the sensory nerves can lead to a painful condition called trigeminal neuralgia. Trigeminal neuralgia affects the trigeminal nerve, one of the largest nerves in the head. The trigeminal nerve is responsible for sensing touch, pain, and temperature in the jaw, gums, forehead, and around the eye area. Trigeminal neuralgia is characterized by very painful, sudden, electric-like spasms in parts of the face. The pain is usually only on one side of the face, often around the eye, cheek, and lower part of the face. It can be triggered by touch, chewing, shaving, or even a light breeze.

Trigeminal nerve damage can also lead to another painful condition called burning mouth syndrome, as the following study confirms. Burning mouth syndrome is often described as a scalding sensation in the tongue, lips, palate, or throughout the mouth.

STUDY

Trigeminal small-fiber sensory neuropathy causes burning mouth syndrome.

Lauria, G., A. Majorana, M. Borgna, R. Lombardi, P. Penza, A. Padovani, P. Sapelli. 2005. *Pain* 115(3):332-7.

"Our study demonstrates that burning mouth syndrome is caused by a trigeminal small-fiber sensory neuropathy and that superficial biopsy of the tongue can be helpful in assessing the diagnosis. These findings shed light into the pathogenesis of this common disorder and could contribute to evaluate targeted therapies in patients."

Sensory nerve damage can also affect hearing and vision. Vision problems, such as blurry vision, double vision, and eye twitching may occur. An eye exam may show damage to the optic nerve, a condition called optic neuritis. Tinnitus, or ringing in the ears, and hearing loss may also result.

CARPAL TUNNEL SYNDROME

Damage to the median nerve, which contains both sensory and motor nerve fibers, could lead to *carpal tunnel syndrome*. The median nerve passes under the carpal ligament that lies across the heel of the hand.

Symptoms include pain, numbness, tingling, burning in the hand, and possible pain from palm to elbow. In the following study researchers found that patients with fibromyalgia had an increased rate (more than 7 times normal) of carpal tunnel syndrome.

STUDY

Evaluation of upper extremity nerve conduction velocities and the relationship between fibromyalgia and carpal tunnel syndrome.

Nacir, B., H. Genc, B. Duvur Cakit, A. Karagoz, H.R. Erdem. 2012. *Arch Med Res.*

“Carpal tunnel syndrome was detected... "in 26 (20.63%) of 126 extremities of 63 patients...We determined an increased rate of carpal tunnel syndrome.”

Subacute combined degeneration of the spinal cord can also lead to a neuropathic pain called a paresthesia, which refers to any abnormal sensation.

According to the National Institutes of Health (NIH), subacute combined degeneration of the spinal cord is *caused* by a vitamin B12 deficiency. The following information is from the NIH.

Subacute Combined Degeneration
National Institutes of Health, 25 June 2009

Subacute combined degeneration of the spinal cord is a disorder that involves weakness, abnormal sensations, mental problems, and vision difficulties.

Causes: Subacute combined degeneration of the spinal cord is caused by a vitamin B12 deficiency.

Subacute combined degeneration primarily affects the spinal cord, but it can also damage the brain, the nerves of the eye, and the peripheral (body) nerves. At first, the disease damages the covering of the nerves (the myelin sheath). It later affects the entire nerve cell.

Symptoms: These symptoms slowly get worse and are usually felt on both sides of the body. Abnormal sensations (tingling and numbness), weakness of the legs, arms, middle of the body, or other areas. Other symptoms include:

- Clumsiness, stiff, or awkward movements
- Unsteady gait and loss of balance
- Change in mental state such as memory problems, irritability, apathy, confusion, or dementia
- Decreased vision
- Depression
- Sleepiness
- Speech impairment (possible)

Low Vitamin B12

In a study published in the *Scandinavian Journal of Rheumatology* researchers found that fibromyalgia and chronic fatigue syndrome patients had *low levels of vitamin B12* and high homocysteine (we will be discussing homocysteine shortly) in their cerebrospinal fluid, where the degenerative changes in the spinal cord are taking place. The researchers also stated they believe that the low vitamin B12 levels found in the cerebrospinal fluid may reflect disruption of the *mechanism of transport* across the blood brain barrier. Here is the conclusion from the study:

> “This study provides convincing preliminary evidence that a high homocysteine level in cerebrospinal fluid is an underlying factor in patients suffering from fibromyalgia and chronic fatigue syndrome. Low vitamin B12 levels in cerebrospinal fluid and possibly low SAMe

levels are implicated as contributing factors. Additional evidence from other studies further support the idea that deficiencies in enzymatic pathways in the brain involving vitamin B12, homocysteine, and folic acid underlie a range of neurological disorders. Deficiencies in these essential biochemical pathways in the brain should be considered by health practitioners in the evaluation of successful interventions for reversing symptoms of fibromyalgia, chronic fatigue syndrome, and other neurological conditions" (Regland,1997).

Vitamin B12 is bound within the dietary proteins we consume in the form of meat, poultry, fish, seafood, dairy, and eggs. Animal protein is the only dietary source of vitamin B12. Protease (pancreatic enzymes that digest dietary proteins) are essential for the proper metabolism of vitamin B12. The following study concludes that *transport and absorption* of vitamin B12 is dependent on the presence of these enzymes. When the abstract speaks of 'R' proteins, it is referring to the amino acids of which proteins are comprised.

STUDY

Cobalamin malabsorption due to nondegradation of R proteins in the human intestine.

Marcoullis G., Y. Parmentier, J.P. Nicolas, M. Jimenez, P. Gerard. 1980. *J Clin Invest*. 66(3):430–440.

"In vivo studies demonstrate that the pancreatic enzymes and the ionic environment in the upper gastrointestinal tract are essential determining factors for transport and absorption of cobalamin in man...These findings confirm the suggestion that the formation of unabsorbable cobalamin complexes may be the reason of impaired vitamin absorption in exocrine pancreatic insufficiency."

CHAPTER 5

Scientific Findings:

Autonomic Nervous System Dysfunction, Orthostatic Hypotension, Overactive Bladder, Dry Eyes and Mouth, and Sleep Apnea

---

AUTONOMIC NERVOUS SYSTEM DYSFUNCTION, orthostatic hypotension, overactive bladder, dry eyes and mouth, and sleep apnea are our next scientific findings.

AUTONOMIC NERVOUS SYSTEM DYSFUNCTION (DYSAUTONOMIA)

Our first study concludes that *autonomic dysfunction* is "inherent" to fibromyalgia (FM).

STUDY

Autonomic dysfunction in fibromyalgia assessed by the Composite Autonomic Symptoms Scale (COMPASS).

Solano, C., A. Martinez, L. Becerril, A. Vargas, J. Figueroa, C. Navarro, C. Ramos-Remus, M. Martinez-Lavin. 2009. *J Clin Rheumatol* 15(4):172-6.

> "Patients with FM have multiple nonpain symptoms related to different expressions of autonomic dysfunction. There is a correlation between a questionnaire that measures FM severity (FIQ) and an autonomic dysfunction questionnaire (COMPASS). Such correlation suggests that autonomic dysfunction is inherent to FM."

The following information on the autonomic nervous system and dysautonomia, which literally means dysregulation of the autonomic nervous system, is from the Merck Manual.

> "The autonomic nervous system is the part of the nervous system that supplies the internal organs, including the blood vessels, stomach, intestine, liver, kidneys, bladder, genitals, lungs, pupils, and muscles of the eye, heart, and sweat, salivary, and digestive glands. The autonomic nervous system controls blood pressure, heart and breathing rates, body temperature, digestion, metabolism (thus affecting body weight), the balance of water and electrolytes (such as sodium and calcium), the production of body fluids (saliva, sweat, and tears), urination, defecation, sexual response, and other processes.
>
> A dysfunction in the autonomic nervous system (dysautonomia) can cause dizziness or light-headedness due to excessive decrease in blood pressure when a person stands (orthostatic hypotension). People may sweat less or not at all and thus become intolerant of heat. The eyes and mouth may become dry. After eating, a person with dysautonomia may feel prematurely full or even vomit because the stomach empties very slowly (gastroparesis).
>
> Some people pass urine involuntarily (urinary incontinence), often because the bladder is overactive. Other people have difficulty emptying the bladder urine retention) because the bladder is underactive. Constipation may occur, or control of bowel movements may be lost. The pupils may not dilate and narrow (constrict) as light changes."

POSTURAL ORTHOSTATIC TACHYCARDIA SYNDROME (POTS)
Orthostatic hypotension, bladder problems, and dry eyes and mouth are all symptoms of autonomic dysfunction. The following study states that *postural orthostatic tachycardia syndrome*, otherwise known as POTS, is one of the most common events experienced by fibromyalgia patients during testing for autonomic dysfunction. Postural orthostatic tachycardia syndrome is characterized by the body's inability to make the necessary adjustments to counteract gravity upon standing.

STUDY

Autonomic dysfunction in fibromyalgia syndrome: postural orthostatic tachycardia.

Staud, R. 2008. *Curr Rheumatol Rep.* 10(6):463-6.

"Although fibromyalgia (FM) syndrome is defined by chronic widespread pain and tenderness, additional symptoms, including disabling fatigue and dizziness, are often reported by patients with this chronic illness...Many important biological functions, such as heart rate, blood pressure, respirations, and bowel function, are tightly regulated by the ANS. However, dysfunction of the ANS is common in FM and often becomes quite apparent after positional changes from supine to upright. Although such positional changes sometimes result in syncope, they are more often associated with palpitations and dizziness. Head-up tilt table testing can be used to evaluate autonomic dysfunction and is frequently helpful for the work-up of FM complaints, including fatigue, dizziness, and palpitations. One of the most common events experienced by FM patients during tilt table testing is postural orthostatic tachycardia syndrome, which is defined as a heart rate increase of more than 30 beats per minute after more than 3 minutes of standing upright."

OVERACTIVE BLADDER

Our next study confirms the association between fibromyalgia syndrome (FMS) and *overactive bladder (OAB)*. Autonomic nervous system dysfunction could also cause the nerves of the bladder to not respond normally to pressure as the bladder fills with urine. This would result in urine staying in the bladder and leading to an increased risk of urinary tract infections.

STUDY

The association between overactive bladder and fibromyalgia syndrome: A community survey.

Chung, J.H., S.A. Kim, B.Y. Choi, H.S. Lee, S.W. Lee, Y.T. Kim, T.Y. Lee, H.S. Moon. 2012. *Neurourol Urodyn.*

"OAB is associated with FMS. Moreover FMS increases with severity of OAB."

DRY EYES AND MOUTH

The autonomic nervous system controls the production of body fluids, such as saliva and tear production. The lack of these body fluids would result in *dry eyes* and *mouth*. Adequate saliva is critical for the prevention of cavities and for the proper digestion of food. In the following study, researchers found decreased tear production in 90% of the fibromyalgia (FM) patients tested.

STUDY

Decreased corneal sensitivity and tear production in fibromyalgia.

Gallar, J., C. Morales, V. Freire, M.C. Acosta, C. Belmonte, J.A. Duran. 2009. *Invest Opthalmol Vis Sci* 50(9):4129-34.

> "The majority (18/20) of patients with FM reported dry eye symptoms, with the ocular dryness score significantly higher in affected subjects than in healthy ones."

The lack of the essential amino acid phenylalanine and vitamin B12 found in fibromyalgia would explain the dysfunction of the autonomic nervous system.

The action of the two branches of the autonomic nervous system is mediated by two neurotransmitters. They are *adrenaline and acetylcholine*. Adrenaline is the predominant sympathetic neurotransmitter, whereas acetylcholine acts in the parasympathetic periphery.

Adrenaline is derived from dopamine, and as we have shown, dopamine is derived from the essential amino acid phenylalanine.

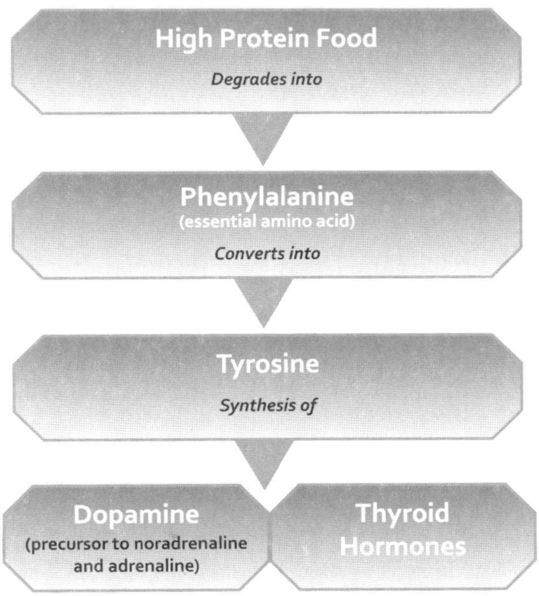

Figure 4.
Diagram demonstrating the production of adrenalin from dopamine and the essential amino acid phenylalanine.

The parasympathetic neurotransmitter is acetylcholine. Acetylcholine is derived from choline. Vitamin B12 and folate are required for the synthesis of choline before becoming acetylcholine.

SLEEP APNEA

Low acetylcholine could also lead to *sleep apnea*. Sleep apnea is defined as the cessation of breathing during sleep. As the following study confirms, sleep apnea is commonly found in patients with fibromyalgia.

STUDY

Sleep-disordered breathing among women with fibromyalgia syndrome.

Shah, M.A., S. Feinberg, E. Krishnan. 2006. *J Clin Rheumatol.* 2006 12(6):277-81.

"A large proportion of women with fibromyalgia in a general rheumatology practice had sleep-disordered breathing... Studies are needed to examine if treatment of the commonly detected sleep apnea will have a beneficial effect on symptoms of fibromyalgia."

Acetylcholine-producing neurons are connected to the part of the brain that controls muscles of the upper airway and tongue, which are involved in sleep apnea. A study published in the journal *Neurology* found that patients with the lowest acetylcholine levels had the most interruptions in their breathing during sleep (Gilman, 2003).

CHAPTER 6

Scientific Findings:

Migraines and Headaches, Elevated Levels of Substance P, Raynaud's Phenomenon, Low Intracellular Magnesium, Elevated Homocysteine, Decreased Levels of Collagen Cross-Linking, Temporomandibular Joint Disorder or TMJ, Mitral Valve Prolapse, Hypermobility, Excess Nitric Oxide, Endometriosis, and an Increased Risk of Cancer

---

OUR NEXT SCIENTIFIC FINDINGS ARE migraines and headaches, elevated levels of substance P, Raynaud's phenomenon, low intracellular magnesium, elevated homocysteine, decreased levels of collagen cross-linking, temporomandibular joint disorder or TMJ, mitral valve prolapse, hypermobility, excess nitric oxide, endometriosis, and an increased risk of cancer.

MIGRAINES AND HEADACHES

Patients with fibromyalgia often suffer with frequent and debilitating *migraines and headaches*. In the following study entitled "Fibromyalgia and headache: an epidemiological study supporting migraine as part of the fibromyalgia syndrome" published in the *Journal of Clinical Rheumatology*, researchers found a high prevalence and significant impact associated with chronic headache in fibromyalgia patients.

STUDY

Fibromyalgia and headache: an epidemiological study supporting migraine as part of the fibromyalgia syndrome.

Marcus, D.A., C. Bernstein, T.E. Rudy. 2005. *Clin Rheumatol.* 24(6):595-601. Epub 2005 May 18.

"In summary, chronic headache was endorsed by 76% of treatment-seeking fibromyalgia patients, with 84% reporting substantial or severe impact from their headaches. Migraine was diagnosed in 63% of fibromyalgia plus headache patients...The high prevalence and significant impact associated with chronic headache in fibromyalgia patients, however, warrants inclusion of a headache assessment as part of the routine evaluation of fibromyalgia patients."

ELEVATED SUBSTANCE P AND RAYNAUD'S PHENOMENON

In our next study, researchers found elevated cerebrospinal fluid (CFS) levels of *substance P* (SP) and a high incidence of *Raynaud's phenomenon* in patients with fibromyalgia. Substance P is a neurotransmitter related to the sensation of pain. Raynaud's phenomenon is a condition in which blood vessels in the fingers or toes react in an exaggerated way (called a vasospasm) to cold or emotional stress. The disruption of blood flow results in cold, numbness, and skin discoloration of the affected parts.

STUDY

Elevated CSF levels of substance P and high incidence of Raynaud phenomenon in patients with fibromyalgia: new features for diagnosis.

Vaerøy, H, R. Helle, O. Førre, E. Kåss, L. Terenius. 2000. *Boll Soc Ital Biol Sper*. 76(1-2):1-4.

"We propose elevated CSF levels of SP and the Raynaud phenomenon as characteristic features for fibromyalgia..."

Low Intracellular Magnesium

In the following study researchers found that patients with fibromyalgia had significantly lower levels of red blood cell (RBC) or *intracellular magnesium*.

STUDY

Magnesium deficiency in fibromyalgia syndrome.

Romano, T.J., J.W. Stiller. 1994. *Journal of Nutritional and Environmental Medicine* Vol. 4, No. 2, Pages 165-167.

"Since patients with either fibromyalgia syndrome (FS) or low magnesium (Mg) levels can have fatigue, sleep disturbance and anxiety, it was necessary to determine if some patients with FS also have low Mg levels... FS patients had significantly lower RBC Mg levels."

Magnesium is needed by the human body to carry out over 300 essential biochemical reactions. According to the National Institutes of Health, magnesium helps maintain normal muscle function and nerve function, keeps the heart rhythm steady, supports a healthy immune system, and keeps bones strong. Magnesium also helps regulate blood sugar levels, promotes normal blood pressure, and is known to be involved in energy metabolism and protein synthesis (National Institutes of Health, 2009).

Because magnesium is active in so many different processes in the body, magnesium deficiency symptoms are varied and can include: insomnia, muscle spasms, muscle twitches and soreness, difficulty swallowing, heart palpitations, extreme fatigue, back aches, chest tightness and difficulty breathing, osteoporosis, and dizziness.

Elevated Homocysteine

In our next study, researchers found that fibromyalgia patients had much higher *homocysteine* levels in their cerebrospinal fluid. The researchers stated, "The mean value of cerebrospinal fluid homocysteine in the patient group was over three times the mean level in the control group, a highly significant difference."

STUDY

Increased concentrations of homocysteine in the cerebrospinal fluid in patients with fibromyalgia and chronic fatigue syndrome.

Regland, B., M. Andersson, L. Abrahamsson, J. Bagby, L.E. Dyrehag, C.G. Gottfries. 1997. *Scand J Rheumatol.* 26(4):301-7.

"The most obvious finding was that, in all the patients, the homocysteine (HCY) levels were increased in the cerebrospinal fluid (CFS)...The mean value of cerebrospinal fluid homocysteine in the patient group was over three times the mean level in the control group, a highly significant difference."

The low levels of vitamin B12 found in patients with fibromyalgia would explain the elevated homocysteine. Homocysteine is derived from the essential amino acid methionine and is used to build and maintain tissue. During normal conditions, excess homocysteine, with the help of vitamin B12, is converted back to methionine or broken down for excretion. The problem arises when the conversion process fails due to the lack of vitamin B12. Homocysteine and vitamin B12 are so closely connected, that currently, one of the most accurate tests for vitamin B12 deficiency is to check for elevated homocysteine levels. If vitamin B12 is deficient, homocysteine goes up.

Homocysteine is a potent nerve and blood vessel toxin that has been found to be approximately 40 times more predictive than cholesterol in assessing risk of cardiovascular disease (Challem, 1996).

Homocysteine damages the cells that line the blood vessels leading to increased rates of cell apoptosis, or cell suicide. These cells are called endothelial cells and they line the entire circulatory system, from the heart to the smallest capillary.

The increased levels of homocysteine would explain the headaches and migraines, elevated levels of substance P, Raynaud's phenomenon, and low intracellular magnesium found in fibromyalgia. Our next study confirms the role of homocysteine in migraines (MA).

STUDY

Homocysteine plasma levels in patients with migraine with aura.

Moschiano. F., D. D'Amico, S. Usai, L. Grazzi, M. Di Stefano, E. Ciusani, N. Erba, G. Bussone. 2008. *Neurol Sci.* 29(Suppl. 1):S173-5.

"We investigated homocysteine plasma levels in 136 MA sufferers and in 117 sex-and age-matched controls. Mean homocysteine plasma levels - as well as the proportion of subjects with hyperhomocysteinaemia - were significantly higher in patients with MA than in healthy controls. Hyperhomocysteinaemia may be a link between MA and ischaemic stroke."

Homocysteine is also linked to Raynaud's phenomenon. The following study, published in the *Journal of Rheumatology*, found that patients with Raynaud's phenomenon (RP) had significantly higher homocysteine concentrations.

STUDY

Elevated homocysteine levels in patients with Raynaud's syndrome.

Levy, Y., J. George, P. Langevitz, D. Harats, R. Doolman, B.A. Sela, Y. Shoenfield. 1999. *J Rheumatol* 26:2383-5.

"Patients with primary and secondary RP had significantly higher homocysteine concentrations compared to healthy individuals."

Our next study shows that homocysteine (HC) causes a depletion of intracellular free magnesium by interfering with magnesium (Mg2+) metabolism. The study concludes, "The present findings are compatible with the hypothesis that an increased serum HC concentration causes abnormal metabolism of Mg2+..."

STUDY

Extracellular magnesium regulates effects of vitamin B_6, B_{12} and folate on homocysteinemia-induced depletion of intracellular free magnesium ions in canine cerebral vascular smooth muscle cells: possible relationship to $[Ca^{2+}]_i$, atherogenesis and stroke.

Wenyan, Li., T. Zheng, J. Wang, B.T. Altura, B.M. Altura. 1999. *Neurosci Lett.* 19 274 (2):83-6 10553943.

"The present findings are compatible with the hypothesis that an increased serum HC concentration causes abnormal metabolism of Mg^{2+} in cerebral VSMC, thus priming these cells for HC-induced atherogenesis, cerebral vasospasm and stroke."

The lack of magnesium would explain the elevated levels of substance P in fibromyalgia. Our next study states, "Magnesium deficiency has been shown to increase substance P."

STUDY

A substance P antagonist increases brain intracellular free magnesium concentration after diffuse traumatic brain injury in rats.

Vink, R. J.J. Donkin, M.I. Cruz, A.J. Nimmo, I. Cernak. 2004. *J Am Coll Nutr.* 23(5):538S-540S.

"Magnesium (Mg) deficiency has been shown to increase substance P ..."

Elevated homocysteine will also explain our next scientific findings of decreased levels of collagen cross-linking, temporomandibular joint disorder or TMJ, mitral valve prolapse, hypermobility, excess nitric oxide, endometriosis, and an increased risk of cancer.

Homocysteine has been shown to interfere with the formation of collagen. In the following study published in *The Journal of Clinical Investigation* the researchers state, "It is concluded that homocysteine interferes with the formation of intermolecular cross-links that help stabilize the collagen macromolecular network."

STUDY

A collagen defect in homocystinuria.

Kang, A.H., R.L. Trelstad. 1973. *J Clin Invest* 52(10):2571-8.

"It is concluded that homocysteine interferes with the formation of intermolecular cross-links that help stabilize the collagen macromolecular network."

DECREASED LEVELS OF COLLAGEN CROSS-LINKING

In the following study researchers found that patients with fibromyalgia have *decreased levels of collagen cross-linking.*

STUDY

Collagen cross-links in fibromyalgia syndrome.

Sprott, H. A. Müller, H. Heine. 1998. *Z Rheumatol.* 57 Suppl 2:52-5.

"To determine whether abnormal collagen metabolism is a characteristic of fibromyalgia, we have analyzed collagen metabolites in the urine and serum of patients with fibromyalgia...Decreased levels of collagen cross-linking may contribute to remodeling of the extracellular matrix..."

TEMPOROMANDIBULAR JOINT DISORDER (TMD)

Collagen disruption could affect the temporomandibular joints, which are made of collagen, and lead to *temporomandibular joint disorder (TMD)*. Our next study concludes that there is a high prevalence of signs and symptoms of temporomandibular dysfunction in fibromyalgia patients.

STUDY

Signs and symptoms of temporomandibular dysfunction in fibromyalgic patients.

Fraga, B.P., E.B. Santos, J.P. Farias Neto, J.C. Macieira, L.J. Quitans Jr., A.S. Onofre, J.M. De Satana, P.R. Martins-Filho, L.R. Bonjardim. 2012. *J Craniofac Surg.* 23(2):615-8.

“Thus, there is a high prevalence of signs and symptoms of TMD in FM patients...”

Mitral Valve Prolapse

Collagen is also a major component of heart valves. A disruption of collagen formation would affect the heart valves and could lead to *mitral valve prolapse*. Mitral valve prolapse is a condition where the mitral valve bulges excessively during the heartbeat. Symptoms may include fatigue, chest pain, heart palpitations, and irregular heartbeat.

Mitral valve prolapse occurs commonly in fibromyalgia. Our next study found that 75% of the fibromyalgia patients tested had mitral valve prolapse.

STUDY

Prevalence of mitral valve prolapse in primary fibromyalgia: a pilot Investigation.

Pellegrino, M.J., D. Van Fossen, C. Gordon, J.M. Ryan, G.W. Waylonis. 1989. *Arch Phys Med Rehabil* 70(7):541-3.

“Mitral valve prolapse was detected in 75%...”

HYPERMOBILITY

Mitral valve prolapse is associated with another condition common in fibromyalgia; *hypermobile joints*. In the following study entitled "Mitral valve prolapse and joint hypermobility: evidence for a systemic connective tissue abnormality" the researchers state, "The results support previous evidence of an association between mitral valve prolapse and benign hypermobility of the joints."

STUDY

Mitral valve prolapse and joint hypermobility: evidence for a systemic connective tissue abnormality?

Pitcher, D., R. Grahame. 1982. *Ann Rheum Dis* 41(4):352-4.

"The results support previous evidence of an association between mitral valve prolapse and benign hypermobility of the joints..."

Collagen makes up 70% of joint cartilage, which would explain the association between mitral valve prolapse and joint hypermobility. The following study confirms the association between fibromyalgia and joint hypermobility.

STUDY

Joint hypermobility in patients with fibromyalgia syndrome.

Acasuso-Díaz, M., E. Collantes-Estévez. 1998. *Arthritis Care Res.*11(1):39-42.

> "The results of this study suggest that joint hypermobility and fibromyalgia are associated. Joint hyperlaxity may play a prominent role in the pathogenesis of pain in fibromyalgia."

Fibromyalgia patients may also develop other conditions caused by unstable joints. These conditions include:

- Joint instability causing frequent sprains, tendinitis, or bursitis when doing activities that would not affect the normal individual
- Early-onset osteoarthritis
- Subluxations or dislocations, especially in the shoulder
- Knee pain
- Back pain, prolapsed discs or spondylolisthesis
- Joints that make clicking noises
- Increased nerve compression disorders, such as carpel tunnel syndrome

Excess Nitric Oxide

Elevated levels of homocysteine can also lead to *excess levels of nitric oxide*. The following study found that nitric oxide synthase (NOS) activity was significantly higher in fibromyalgia patients. Nitric oxide synthase produces nitric oxide.

STUDY

Arginase, NOS activities, and clinical features in fibromyalgia patients.

Cimen, O.B., M.Y. Cimen, Y. Yapici, H. Camdeviren. 2009. *Pain Med.* 10(5):813-8.

> "We found that NOS activity was significantly higher..."

Nitric oxide is an important "messenger molecule" in the body. It can be either beneficial or toxic, depending on the body's ability to properly regulate it. The beneficial properties of nitric oxide are diverse. It is a key ingredient in many erectile dysfunction products because it stimulates penile blood flow. It helps the immune system fight off infection and cancer cells, and in the brain it helps cells communicate properly.

In our blood vessels, nitric oxide can "signal" the surrounding arterial tissues and cause them to relax. This will lower blood pressure and expand narrow blood vessels leading to improved circulation. Increased blood flow will bring more oxygen to our cells and tissues and this will, in turn, lead to more energy and better brain function.

An excess of nitric oxide, though, will react with O2-, a potent free radical, and form peroxynitrite, a powerful oxidant, as the following study shows. Peroxynitrite is known to damage cells through multiple mechanisms.

STUDY

Nitric oxide, superoxide, and peroxynitrite: the good, the bad, and ugly.

Beckman, J.S., W.H. Koppenol. 1996. *Am J Physiol.* 271(5 Pt 1):C1424-37.

"The direct toxicity of nitric oxide is modest but is greatly enhanced by reacting with superoxide to form peroxynitrite (ONOO-)."

The following study found that elevated levels of homocysteine significantly increased nitric oxide production (150% of the control), which then resulted in the formation of peroxynitrite.

STUDY

Hyperhomcysteinemia activates NF-kappaB and inducible nitric oxide synthase in the kidney.

> Zhang, F., Y.L. Siow, O. K. 2004. *Kidney Int.* 65(4):1327-38.
>
> "Increased nitric oxide production (150% of the control) resulted in peroxynitrite formation in these kidneys. Hyperhomocysteinemia alone can activate NF-kappaB and hence induce iNOS-mediated nitric oxide production in the kidney leading to increased peroxynitrite formation. This may represent one of the mechanisms for renal dysfunction in hyperhomocysteinemia."

An excess of nitric oxide can also interfere with the body's ability to properly regulate the development of new blood vessels or angiogenesis. In the research paper entitled "Nitric oxide and angiogenesis" the researchers state, "Elevation of NOS (nitric oxide synthase) activity in correlation with angiogenesis and tumor progression has been extensively reported in experimental and human tumors" (Cooke, 2002).

The development of new blood vessels is a relatively infrequent event in adults. In women, angiogenesis is active a few days each month as new blood vessels form in the lining of the uterus during the menstrual cycle. Also, angiogenesis is necessary for the repair or regeneration of tissue during wound healing. Slow wound healing is often a feature of fibromyalgia.

By interfering with nitric oxide (NO), homocysteine can prevent wounds from healing normally. The study entitled "Homocysteine and impaired wound heal" states, "Ongoing experimental and clinical wound healing studies have now clearly established NO as a critical mediator of normal tissue repair. Angiogenesis, granulation tissue formation, epidermal migration, collagen deposition, and microvascular homeostasis are significant vulnerary processes, critical to normal wound repair, that are regulated by NO production and bioactivity...Homocysteine antagonizes NO production via multiple pathways..."(Boykin, 2005).

Nitric oxide regulates a protein called vascular endothelial growth factor (VEGF) that stimulates angiogenesis. Without proper instruction from VEGF, endothelial cells (cells that line the blood vessels) can be stimulated to proliferate and migrate. The following study states that nitric oxide plays a critical role in VEGF-induced angiogenesis.

STUDY

Predominant role of endothelial nitric oxide synthase in vascular endothelial growth factor-induced angiogenesis and vascular permeability.

Fukumura, D., T. Gohongi, A. Kadambi, Y. Izumi, J. Ang, C.O. Yun, D.G. Buerk, P.L. Huang, R.K. Jain. 2001. *P Natl Acad Sci. USA* 98(5):2604-9.

"Nitric oxide (NO) plays a critical role in vascular endothelial growth factor (VEGF)-induced angiogenesis and vascular hyperpermeability."

ENDOMETRIOSIS

Angiogenesis has long been a recognized feature of *endometriosis*. Endometriosis is defined as the growth of endometrial tissue outside the uterine cavity. This excess growth pattern can lead to diverse symptoms, such as pelvic pain, infertility, and heavy bleeding. According to the National Institutes of Health (NIH) there is a "strong association" between endometriosis and fibromyalgia (NIH, 2002).

Our next studies confirm the involvement of excess nitric oxide and VEGF in endometriosis.

STUDY

Nitric oxide synthesis is increased in the endometrial tissue of women with endometriosis.

Wu, M.Y., K.H. Chao, J.H. Yang, T.H. Lee, Y.S. Yang, H.N. Ho. 2003. *Hum Reprod 18*(12):2688-74.

"Greater amounts of NO and NOS are present in the endometrial tissues of women with endometriosis."

STUDY

Increased nitric oxide in peritoneal fluid from women with idiopathic infertility and endometriosis.

Dong, M., Y. Shi, Q. Cheng, M. Hao. 2001. *J Repro Med* 46(10):887-91.

"To verify whether nitric oxide in peritoneal fluid is associated with endometriosis and infertility...An increased peritoneal level of nitric oxide is a common alteration in endometriosis, endometriosis-associated infertility and idiopathic infertility and may be associated with the pathogenesis of these diseases."

STUDY

Vascular endothelial growth factor (VEGF) concentrations are elevated in peritoneal fluid of women with endometriosis.

McLaren J, A. Prentice, D.S. Charnock-Jones, S.K. Smith. 1996. *Hum Reprod*. 11(1):220-3.

"Active endometriosis is characterized by hypervascularization both within and surrounding the implant; therefore the presence of angiogenic factors in the peritoneal environment would be of great importance. Vascular endothelial growth factor (VEGF) is a potent angiogenic factor involved in both physiological and pathological angiogenesis. We sought to determine if VEGF was present in the peritoneal fluid of women with and without endometriosis, and to establish if differences exist between these groups. VEGF was present in all patients sampled. The fluid from patients with endometriosis contained significantly greater amounts of VEGF than controls...We suggest that elevated levels of VEGF in the peritoneal fluid of patients with endometriosis may be critical in the pathogenesis of endometriosis."

At this point, a logical conclusion would be that there may be a correlation to the angiogenesis found in endometriosis, due to the improper regulation of vascular endothelial growth factor by nitric oxide, and cancer. In fact, women with endometriosis and fibromyalgia are at a higher risk of developing certain cancers, such as breast cancer, as the following studies demonstrate.

STUDY

The risk of cancer and the role of parity among women with endometriosis.

Melin, A., P. Sparén , A. Bergqvist. 2007. *Hum Reprod.* 22(11):3021-6. Epub 2007 Sep 13.

"Endometriosis was associated with elevated risks for endocrine tumours... ovarian cancer... renal cancer... thyroid cancer... brain tumours... malignant melanoma... and breast cancer... Women with endometriosis have an increased risk for several malignancies. The increased risks do not seem to be related to parity." (Parity is the number of times a female has given birth.)

INCREASED RISK OF CANCER

The following study found a substantial *increased risk of cancer* in patients with widespread body pain. In regards to this finding the researchers stated, "Widespread body pain is the cardinal symptom of fibromyalgia syndrome."

STUDY

Association of widespread body pain with an increased risk of cancer and reduced cancer survival: a prospective, population-based study.

McBeth, J., A.J. Silman, G.J. Macfarlane. 2003. *Arthritis Rheum.* 48(6):1686-92.

"This study has demonstrated that widespread pain reported in population surveys is associated with a substantial subsequent increased incidence of cancer and reduced cancer survival...Widespread body pain is the cardinal symptom of the fibromyalgia syndrome."

Are nitric oxide and vascular endothelial growth factor linked to cancer also? Studies confirm that this is indeed the case. For instance, the following study found that nitric oxide and vascular endothelial growth factor are involved in breast cancer and that this involvement correlates with "metastasis and poor prognosis."

STUDY

Nitric oxide in breast cancer: induction of vascular endothelial growth factor-C and correlation with metastasis and poor prognosis.

Nakamura, Y., H. Yasuoka, M. Tsuijmoto, K. Yoshidome, M. Nakamura, K. Kakudo. 2006. *Clin Cancer Res* 12(4):1201-7.

"Our data showed a role for NO in stimulating VEGF-C expression in vitro. Formation of its biomarker nitrotyrosine was also correlated with VEGF-C expression and lymph node metastasis."

If the link between fibromyalgia, endometriosis, and cancer is an excess of nitric oxide, due to elevated levels of homocysteine, then we should find increased levels of homocysteine in breast cancer and endometriosis, just as we have found in fibromyalgia.

The following study on homocysteine and metastatic breast cancer found that women with metastatic disease had significantly higher homocysteine concentrations.

STUDY

Raised plasma homocysteine levels in women with metastatic breast cancer.

Makris, A., H. Cladd, R.J. Burcombe, J.M. Smith, M. Makris. 2001. *Proc Am Soc Clin Oncol.* 20: Abstract 179.

"Women with metastatic disease had significantly higher plasma homocysteine concentrations compared to controls...We conclude that hyperhomocysteinaemia is common in women with metastatic breast cancer."

In our next study the researchers found that elevated homocysteine (Hcy) levels were significantly linked to an increased risk of breast cancer and that the increased cancer risk was observed in both premenopausal and post-menopausal women. In addition, the researchers felt the link was so strong that homocysteine could be considered a metabolic risk factor for breast cancer.

STUDY

Plasma homocysteine as a metabolic risk factor for breast cancer: findings from a case-control study in Taiwan.

Chou, Y.C., M.S. Lee, M.H. Wu, H.L. Shih, T. Yang, C.P. Yu, J.C. Yu, C.A. Sun. 2007. *Breast Cancer Res Tr.* 101(2):199-205.

"Elevated plasma Hcy levels were significantly linked to increased risk of breast cancer... Moreover, a similar pattern of enhanced breast cancer risk at higher plasma Hcy levels was observed in both pre-menopausal and post-menopausal women. The current study results seem to suggest a possibility that the plasma Hcy levels could be a metabolic risk factor for breast cancer."

The following study confirms elevated levels of homocysteine in endometriosis.

STUDY

Impact of folate and homocysteine metabolism on human reproductive health.

Oxford Journals Press. Hum. Reprod. Update (2007).

"Follicular fluid homocysteine concentration was significantly higher in women with endometriosis when compared with patients having unexplained infertility."

Of course, angiogenesis is only one component of cancer, but it is an important component. Cancer spreads to other locations in the body by metastasis. In large measure, it is this ability to spread to other tissues and organs that makes cancer a potentially life-threatening disease. According to the National Cancer Institute, angiogenesis is necessary for cancerous tumors to grow and spread. They state: "Before the 1960s, cancer researchers believed that the blood supply reached tumors simply because pre-existing blood vessels dilated. But later experiments showed that angiogenesis--the growth of the new blood vessels--is necessary for cancerous tumors to keep growing and spreading. Without angiogenesis, tumor growth stops" (National Cancer Institute, 2005).

The National Cancer Institute also states that vascular endothelial growth factor (VEGF), along with another protein called basic fibroblast growth factor, appear to be the most important for sustaining tumor growth (National Cancer Institute, 2005). The identification of the reason why VEGF is being dysregulated could be an extremely important factor in reducing the possibility of someone with fibromyalgia succumbing to cancer.

CHAPTER 7

Scientific Findings:

Elevated Tumor Necrosis Factor (TNF), Allodynia, Excessive Daytime Sleepiness, Chronic Urticaria, Allergies, and Inflammatory Bowel Disease

OUR NEXT FINDINGS ARE elevated tumor necrosis factor (TNF), allodynia, excessive daytime sleepiness, chronic urticaria, allergies, and inflammatory bowel disease.

ELEVATED TUMOR NECROSIS FACTOR (TNF)

In the following study researchers found that fibromyalgia (FM) patients had higher levels than normal of a cytokine called *tumor necrosis factor (TNF)*.

STUDY

Cytokine patterns in fibromyalgia and their correlation with clinical manifestations.

Bazzichi, L., A. Rossi, G. Massimetti, G. Giannaccini, T. Giuliano, F. De Feo, A. Ciapparelli, L. Dell'Osso, S. Bombardieri. 2007. *Clin Exp Rheumatol*. 25(2):225-30.

> "Higher levels of ...TNF-alpha were found in FM patients than in controls. Significant correlations between the biochemical parameters and clinical data were found."

Tumor necrosis factor (TNF) is part of the body's inflammatory immune system. Cells of the immune system produce proteins called cytokines. There are different types of cytokines-including TNF. Cytokines do amazing things to fight off infection. Much like homocysteine though, if TNF is not controlled, it is capable of doing a great deal of damage to the body.

Elevated TNF will produce such symptoms as malaise, night sweats, sore throat, swollen glands, and low-grade fevers. Elevated TNF may be the reason why some patients with fibromyalgia say they feel as if they always have the flu. This is the same part of the immune system that would be activated if you actually did have the flu.

ALLODYNIA

Elevated tumor necrosis factor can also lead to a painful condition experienced by fibromyalgia patients known as *allodynia*. Allodynia is pain, generally on the skin, and is an exaggerated response to stimuli that normally doesn't cause pain. Someone with allodynia may experience pain from a light touch or fabric brushing against the skin. It is often described as a burning sensation.

Specialized nerve cells, called nociceptors, are the cells involved in allodynia. Nociceptors sense information involving skin pain and temperature and transmit it to the spinal cord. Tumor necrosis factor binds to receptors expressed on nociceptors and leads to the exaggerated pain response found in allodynia (Wei, 2007).

EXCESSIVE DAYTIME SLEEPINESS

Tumor necrosis factor is also involved in the sleep/wake cycle in the body, which is regulated by the Hypocretin system. An impairment in the Hypocretin system could result in narcolepsy, which is a chronic neurological disorder caused by the brain's inability to regulate sleep-wake cycles normally. Research has shown that fibromyalgia patients have disturbance of sleep that is similar to narcolepsy (Spitzer, 2010). *Excessive daytime sleepiness*, which is the main symptom of narcolepsy, is often experienced by patients with fibromyalgia (Himmerich, 2006).

In the following study the researchers found that narcoleptic patients had increased plasma levels of TNF which was suggestive of a "functional alteration" of the TNF cytokine system.

STUDY

Plasma levels of tumor necrosis factor α and soluble tumor necrosis factor receptors in patients with narcolepsy.

Himmerich, H., P.A. Beitinger, F. Stephany Fulda, R. Wehrle, J. Linseisen, G. Wolfram, S. Himmerich, K. Gedrich, T.C. Wetter, T. Pollmächer. 2006. *Arch Intern Med.* 166(16):1739-1743.

"Narcolepsy is a disabling sleep disorder characterized by excessive daytime sleepiness, cataplexy, hypnagogic hallucinations, and sleep paralysis. Recent studies suggest that the immune system might play a pathogenic role pointing to a possible involvement of inflammatory cytokines...Narcoleptic patients show increased plasma levels of sTNF-R p75, suggesting a functional alteration of the TNF-α cytokine system, further corroborating a possible pathogenic role of the immune system in this sleep disorder."

Our next study states that TNF regulates the Hypocretin system. Therefore, a functional alteration in TNF would impair the Hypocretin system. This would explain the excessive daytime sleepiness often experienced by patients with fibromyalgia.

STUDY

Tumor necrosis factor-alpha regulates the Hypocretin system via mRNA degradation and ubiquitination.

Zhan, S., G.Q. Cai, A. Zheng, Y. Wang, J. Jia, H. Fang, Y. Yang, M. Hu, Q. Ding. 2011. *Biochim Biophys Acta.* 1812(4):565-71.

"Recent studies recognize that Hypocretin system (also known as Orexin) plays a critical role in sleep/wake disorders and feeding behaviors. However, little is known about the regulation of the Hypocretin system. It is also known that tumor necrosis factor alpha (TNF-α) is involved in the regulation of sleep/wake cycle... These studies demonstrate that TNF-α can impair the function of the Hypocretin system..."

CHRONIC URTICARIA (HIVES)

Tumor necrosis factor is also implicated in *chronic urticaria (hives)*, which is associated with fibromyalgia, as the following study confirms.

STUDY

Chronic urticaria is usually associated with fibromyalgia syndrome.

Torresani,C., S. Bellafiore, G. De Panfilis. 2009. *Acta Derm Venereol.* 89(4):389-92.

"Chronic urticaria may thus be viewed in many patients, as a consequence of fibromyalgia syndrome..."

As the following study states, the primary cell involved in chronic urticaria is likely the mast cell, which releases tumor necrosis factor.

STUDY

Treatment of refractory chronic urticaria with tumor necrosis factor–alfa inhibitors.

Wilson, L.H., Eliason, M.J., Leiferman, K.M., Hull, C.M., Powell, D.L. 2011. *Journal of the American Academy of Dermatology* Volume 64, Issue 6 , Pages 1221-1222.

"The pathogenic mechanisms of chronic urticaria are not well understood, but the primary effector cell is likely the mast cell. Activated mast cells release mediators, including tumor necrosis factor–alfa (TNF-α), that recruit other immune cells and play a role in perpetuating an urticarial response. TNF-α is known to exist preformed in mast cells and to be newly synthesized upon mast cell activation. Several preclinical investigations have shown an upregulation of TNF-α in patients with chronic urticaria."

Allergies

Mast cells and tumor necrosis factor are also involved in *allergies*. In the following study, researchers found that about 50% of the fibromyalgia (FB) patients studied had symptoms of allergy.

STUDY

The lymphocyte phenotype in patients with primary fibromyalgia.

Samborski, W., J.K. Lacki, K.E. Wiktorowicz. 1996. *Ups J Med Sci.* 101(3):251-6.

"Moreover, the symptoms to allergy has been found in about 50% of our patients. Taken together the data thus far obtained present a coexistence of symptoms of allergy and FB."

As the next study states, mast cell-derived tumor necrosis factor is "essential" for allergic airway disease.

STUDY

Mast cell-derived tumor necrosis factor is essential for allergic airway disease.

Reuter, S., A. Heinz, M. Sieren, R. Wiewrodt, E.W. Gelfand, M. Stassen, R. Buhl, C. Taube. 2008. *Eur Respir J.* 31(4):773-82. Epub 2007 Dec 19.

"The present results demonstrate the significance of mast cells in the development of airway disease and highlight the importance of mast cell-derived tumor necrosis factor in these responses."

Recurrent aphthous ulceration (RAU) or canker sores, which are often experienced by patients with fibromyalgia, can also be attributed to tumor necrosis factor.

The study entitled "Salivary interleukin-6 and tumor necrosis factor-alpha in patients with recurrent aphthous ulceration" states that, "Recurrent aphthous ulceration (RAU) is a well-known oral disease which seems to be mediated principally by the immune system" (Boras, 2006). The researchers found significant differences in salivary tumor necrosis factor between healthy controls and patients with acute RAU. No differences in salivary interleukin-6 between the groups could be found.

INFLAMMATORY BOWEL DISEASE (IBD)

An excess of TNF can also lead to *inflammatory bowel disease (IBD),* or Crohn's disease and ulcerative colitis. In the following study, researchers concluded that fibromyalgia is common in IBD, particularly Crohn's disease.

STUDY

Fibromyalgia in inflammatory bowel disease.

Buskila, D, L.R. Odes, L. Neumann, H.S. Odes. 1999. *J Rheumatol.* 26(5):1167-71.

"FM is common in IBD, particularly Crohn's disease."

One of the drugs used to treat Crohns's disease is Humira®. The Humira® website states, "Many patients with Crohn's disease produce too much of a protein called tumor necrosis factor (TNF) in their body. This excess attacks the intestines and other parts of the gastrointestinal (GI) tract, and can cause them to become inflamed. This can result in the pain, diarrhea, and other symptoms of Crohn's disease. Humira® belongs to a class of biologics known as TNF blockers" (Humira.com).

So, why is there an excess of TNF? What is responsible for keeping it within normal limits and degrading it when necessary? As the following study shows, the degradation and inactivation of TNF is performed by pancreatic proteases.

STUDY

Degradation and inactivation of plasma tumor necrosis factor-alpha by pancreatic proteases in experimental acute pancreatitis.

Alsfasser G., B. Antoniu, S.P. Thayer, A.L. Warshaw, C. Fernández-del Castillo. 2005. *Pancreatology* 5(1):37-43.

"Our study demonstrates degradation and inactivation of TNF-alpha by pancreatic proteases."

Protease specifically regulate cytokines, such as TNF, as our next study confirms.

STUDY

Neutrophil serine proteases fine-tune the inflammatory response.

Pham, C.T.N. 2008. *Int J Biochem Cell Biol.* 40(6-7):1317-1333.

"However, studies over the past several years indicate that neutrophil serine proteases may also be key regulators of the inflammatory response. Neutrophil serine proteases specifically process and release chemokines, cytokines, and growth factors, thus modulating their biological activity. In addition, neutrophil serine proteases activate and shed specific cell surface receptors, which can ultimately prolong or terminate cytokine-induced responses."

CHAPTER 8

Scientific Findings:

Low GABA, Anxiety, Association with ADHD, Sound Sensitivity, Severe Premenstrual Syndrome (PMS), Elevated Glutamate, Depression, Bipolar Disorder, Increased Risk of Suicide, Irritable Bowel Syndrome, Interstitial Cystitis, Inflammation of the Fascia, and Increased Kynurenine Pathway Activity

---

OUR NEXT FINDINGS ARE low GABA, anxiety, association with ADHD, sound sensitivity, severe premenstrual syndrome (PMS), elevated glutamate, depression, bipolar disorder, increased risk of suicide, irritable bowel syndrome, interstitial cystitis, inflammation of the fascia, and increased kynurenine pathway activity.

Low GABA

In the following study the researchers found that fibromyalgia (FM) patients had significantly *lower levels of GABA* in a section of the brain.

STUDY

Reduced insular γ-aminobutyric acid in fibromyalgia.

Foerster, B.R., M. Petrou, R.A. Edden, P.C. Sundgren, T. Schmidt-Wilcke, S.E. Lowe, S.E. Harte, D.J. Clauw, R.E. Harris. 2012. *Arthritis Rheum*. Feb;64(2):579-83.

"GABA levels in the right anterior insula were significantly lower in FM patients compared with healthy controls...Diminished inhibitory neurotransmission resulting from lower concentrations of GABA within the right anterior insula may play a role in the pathophysiology of FM and other central pain syndromes."

ANXIETY

GABA (gamma-aminobutyric acid) is the major inhibitory neurotransmitter in the brain. Excitation in the brain must be balanced with inhibition. Too much excitation can lead to anxiety, insomnia, impulsivity, inability to focus attention, and even seizures. Anti-anxiety medications, such as benzodiazepines and barbiturates, work by binding to GABA receptors to increase its inhibitory effect and relieve anxiety. The significantly lower levels of GABA found in fibromyalgia patients would clearly explain our next scientific finding-*anxiety.* In the following study the researchers found that 50% of the patients with fibromyalgia suffered from anxiety.

STUDY

An evaluation of anxiety and depression symptoms in fibromyalgia.

dos Santos, E.B., L.J. Quintans Junior, B.P. Fraga, J.C. Macieira, L.R. Bonjardim. 2012. *Rev Esc Enferm USP.* 46(3):590-6.

"The frequency of anxiety and depression symptoms was, respectively, 50% and 86% for individuals with fibromyalgia...Anxiety and depression were frequent symptoms among patients with fibromyalgia."

ADHD

Researchers from our next study concluded that fibromyalgia and *ADHD* share a common etiopathological (cause of disease) mechanism.

STUDY

High frequency of childhood ADHD history in women with fibromyalgia.

Reyero, F., G. Ponce, R. Rodriguez-Jimenez, P. Fernandez-Dapica, D. Taboada, V. Martin, M. Navio, M.A. Jimenez-Arriero, J. Hoenicka, T. Palomo. 2011. *Eur Psychiatry*. 26(8):482-3. Epub 2010 Jul 10.

"Our data suggest that Fibromyalgia and ADHD have some common etiopathological mechanism."

Low levels of GABA are also associated with attention-deficit/hyperactivity disorder (ADHD), as the following study from Johns Hopkins University School of Medicine confirms.

STUDY

Reduced GABA concentration in attention-deficit/hyperactivity disorder.

Edden, R.A., D. Crocetti, H. Zhu, D.L. Gilbert, S.H. Mostofsky. 2012. *Arch Gen Psychiatry*. 69(7):750-3.

"Attention-deficit/hyperactivity disorder (ADHD) is a developmental disorder characterized by a deficit in behavioral inhibition. Recent evidence also suggests a deficit in cortical inhibition via the GABA (γ-aminobutyric acid)-ergic system…GABA concentration is reduced in children with ADHD compared with typically developing control subjects. Our finding of reduced GABA concentration in ADHD is concordant with recently reported deficits in short intracortical inhibition in ADHD and suggests a GABAergic deficit in ADHD.”

SOUND SENSITIVITY

Sensitivity to sound is our next finding. In the following study the researchers found that patients with fibromyalgia (FM) displayed significantly greater sensitivity to all levels of auditory stimulation and were also more sensitive to everyday sounds.

STUDY

A psychophysical study of auditory and pressure sensitivity in patients with fibromyalgia and healthy controls.

Geisser, M.E., J.M. Glass, L.D. Rajcevska, D.J. Clauw, D.A. Williams, P.R. Kileny, R.H. Gracely. 2008. *J Pain*.

“Participants with FM displayed significantly greater sensitivity to all levels of auditory stimulation… FM patients also were more sensitive to everyday sounds…”

The sensitivity to sound found in patients with fibromyalgia can also be attributed to low GABA. The following study found that blocking GABA increased sensitivity to sound.

STUDY

Blocking GABAergic inhibition increases sensitivity to sound motion cues in the inferior colliculus.

McAlpine, D. and A.R. Palmer. 2002. *The Journal of Neuroscience* 22(4):1443–1453.

"These results indicate that GABAergic inhibition strongly influences the context-dependent processing of low-frequency binaural signals in the IC."

Severe Premenstrual Syndrome (PMS)

Many patients with fibromyalgia also suffer with *severe premenstrual syndrome* (PMS) (Amital, 2010). Premenstrual syndrome occurs when there is a drop in progesterone levels just prior to the start of the menstrual period. Common symptoms of PMS are anxiety, depression, and irritability. In the following study the researchers found that patients with premenstrual dysphoric disorder, or severe PMS, had low levels of GABA.

STUDY

Low plasma gamma-aminobutyric acid levels during the late luteal phase of women with premenstrual dysphoric disorder.

Halbreich, U., F. Petty, K. Yonkers, G.L. Kramer, A.J. Rush, K.W. Bibi. 1996. *Am J Psychiatry.* 153(5):718-20.

"In women with premenstrual dysphoric disorder... plasma GABA levels decreased from the nonsymptomatic, mid-follicular phase to the symptomatic, late luteal phase."

The following additional study from Yale University School of Medicine confirms the connection between low GABA and premenstrual dysphoric disorder "PMDD".

STUDY

Cortical gamma-aminobutyric acid levels across the menstrual cycle in healthy women and those with premenstrual dysphoric disorder: a proton magnetic resonance spectroscopy study.

Epperson, C.N., K. Haga, G.F. Mason, E. Sellers, R. Gueorguieva, W. Zhang, E. Weiss, D.L. Rotham. 2002. *Arch Gen Psychiatry*. 59(9):851-8.

"These data strongly suggest that the GABAergic system is substantially modulated by menstrual cycle phase in healthy women and those with PMDD. Furthermore, they raise the possibility of disturbances in cortical GABA neuronal function and modulation by neuroactive steroids as potentially important contributors to the pathogenesis of PMDD."

The declining levels of progesterone just prior to the onset of the menstrual cycle are responsible for the low levels of GABA and resulting symptoms found in PMS. The progesterone metabolite allopregnanolone is a potent modulator of GABA receptors. In the following study researchers found that withdrawal from progesterone supplementation increased anxiety and seizure susceptibility due to declining levels of this potent GABA-modulatory metabolite.

STUDY

Progesterone withdrawal reduces paired-pulse inhibition in rat hippocampus: dependence on GABA(A) receptor alpha4 subunit upregulation.

Hsu, F.C. and S.S. Smith. 2003. *J Neurophysiol*. 89(1):186-98.

> "Withdrawal from the endogenous steroid progesterone (P) after chronic administration increases anxiety and seizure susceptibility via declining levels of its potent GABA-modulatory metabolite..."

Elevated Glutamate

While GABA is the major inhibitory neurotransmitter in the brain, glutamate is the major excitatory neurotransmitter. As our next study confirms, fibromyalgia patients have significantly *higher levels of glutamate* in their cerebrospinal fluid. Glutamate mediates central sensitization (Gudin, 2004). Central sensitization is a condition of the nervous system that is associated with the development and maintenance of chronic pain. The following study discusses the association between central sensitization and the "tender points" found in fibromyalgia, due to the increase in glutamate levels. Central sensitization can lead to heightened sensitivities across all senses, not just the sense of touch. Fibromyalgia patients often report other sensitivities, such as those to light and odors.

Research shows that central sensitization is also associated with chronic low back pain (O'Neill, 2007) and chronic neck pain (Chua, 2011), both of which are associated with fibromyalgia. A recent study found 28 percent of women with chronic low back pain also met the criteria for fibromyalgia (Nordeman, 2012).

The following study also discusses the association between elevated glutamate and migraines. The significantly higher levels of glutamate, along with the damaging effects of homocysteine on the blood vessels, would clearly explain the comorbidity of chronic migraine with fibromyalgia.

STUDY

Cerebrospinal fluid glutamate levels in chronic migraine.

Peres, M.F., E. Zukerman, C.A. Senne Soares, E.O. Alonso, B.F. Santos, M.H. Faulhaber. 2004. *Cephalalgia* 24(9):735-9.

> "Both preclinical and clinical data link glutamate to the migraine pathophysiology. Altered plasma, platelets and cerebrospinal (CSF) glutamate levels have been reported in migraine patients. Chronic migraine is comorbid with several conditions. It has been recently shown chronic migraine comorbidity with fibromyalgia...CSF glutamate demonstrated significantly higher levels in patients with fibromyalgia compared to those without fibromyalgia...Tender points, the hallmark of fibromyalgia... is probably mediated by central sensitization, with increase in CSF glutamate levels."

DEPRESSION AND BIPOLAR DISORDER

Depression and *bipolar disorder* are commonly associated with fibromyalgia. The following study from the Cleveland Clinic found that just over 25% of patients with fibromyalgia had symptoms of bipolar disorder and over 78% of the fibromyalgia patients were clinically depressed. In addition, the researchers state that over 52% of the fibromyalgia patients reported daytime sleepiness.

STUDY

Fibromyalgia and bipolar disorder: a potential problem?

Wilke, W.S., C.E. Gota, D.J. Muzina. 2010. *Bipolar Disord.* 12(5):514-20.

> "A quarter of the fibromyalgia subjects, 25.19%, had a positive screen for bipolar disorder... 78.12% were clinically depressed... and 52.13% reported daytime sleepiness."

INCREASED RISK OF SUICIDE

Fibromyalgia (FM) is also associated with an *increased risk of suicide*, as the following study confirms.

STUDY

Suicide attempts and risk of suicide in patients with fibromyalgia: a survey in Spanish patients.

Calandre, E.P., J.S. Vilchez, R. Molina-Barea, M. Isabel Tovar, J.M. Garcia-Leiva, J. Hildago, C.M. Rodriquez-Lopez, F. Rico-Villadermoros. 2011. *Rheumatology.*

"FM is associated with an increased risk of suicide and suicide attempts. Suicidal behavior seems to be related with the global severity of the disease."

Irritable Bowel Syndrome

Patients with fibromyalgia are also likely to have *irritable bowel syndrome (IBS).* The following study found that 70% of the fibromyalgia patients tested had IBS, which led the researchers to suggest that both conditions share a common pathogenetic mechanism.

STUDY

Primary fibromyalgia and the irritable bowel syndrome: different expressions of a common pathogenetic process.

Veale, D., G. Kavanagh, J.F. Fielding, O. Fitzgerald. 1991. *Br J Rheumatol.* 30(3):220-2.

"Results indicate that 70% ... of the PFM patients had IBS and 65% ... of the IBS patients had PFM. In conclusion, these results indicate that PFM and IBS frequently coexist. A common pathogenetic mechanism for both conditions is therefore suggested."

INTERSTITIAL CYSTITIS

Our next study confirms the association of a chronic bladder disorder called *interstitial cystitis* with fibromyalgia. Interstitial cystitis is characterized by pain in the bladder and pelvic region, typically accompanied by urinary urgency and frequency.

STUDY

Interstitial cystitis/painful bladder syndrome and associated medical conditions with an emphasis on irritable bowel syndrome, fibromyalgia and chronic fatigue syndrome.

Nickel, J.C., D.A. Tripp, M. Pontari, R. Moldwin, R. Mayer, L.K. Carr, R. Doggweiler, C.C. Yang, N. Mishra, J. Nordling. 2010. *J Urol.* 184(4):1358-63. Epub 2010 Aug 17.

"Irritable bowel syndrome, fibromyalgia and chronic fatigue syndrome are more prevalent in patients with interstitial cystitis/painful bladder syndrome than in asymptomatic control subjects, and result in significant impact."

Myofascial pain syndrome, which involves muscle pain with specific "trigger" or "tender" points, is often associated with fibromyalgia. Myofascial means "fascia related to the muscles". The fascia (connective tissue that covers the muscles) is as sensitive to pain as skin. In addition to covering the muscles, the fascia envelops and intertwines with organs, bones, and joints. It also enters into the muscles themselves.

Inflamed or damaged fascia can tighten and contract, putting painful pressure on nerves and muscles, causing many different types of pain. Myofascial pain is often described as aching, burning, stinging, or stabbing. It can occur in the neck, shoulders, jaw, low back, and arms and legs. Damaged fascia can also lead to muscle stiffness and weakness and a reduced range of motion in the affected parts.

Inflammation of the Fascia

In our next study, done at Oregon Health and Science University, researchers found evidence for dysfunction of the fascia in fibromyalgia. In addition, the researchers stated that the *inflammation found in the fascia* of the patients with fibromyalgia is similar to that described in conditions such as plantar fasciitis. Plantar fasciitis, which is often reported in fibromyalgia patients, is inflammation of the thick band of connective tissue called the plantar fascia. The plantar fascia runs along the sole from the bottom of the heal bone to the toes.

STUDY

Fascia: A missing link in our understanding of the pathology of fibromyalgia.

Liptan, G.L. 2010. *J Bodyw Mov Ther.* Jan;14(1):3-12.

"However, there is some evidence for dysfunction of the intramuscular connective tissue, or fascia, in fibromyalgia."

Increased Kynurenine Pathway Activity

Low GABA, elevated glutamate, depression, bipolar disorder, increased risk of suicide, irritable bowel syndrome, interstitial cystitis, and inflammation of the fascia can all be explained by the abnormal metabolism of the essential amino acid tryptophan through what is known as the *kynurenine pathway*.

The body has alternate pathways to metabolize the essential amino acid tryptophan. In one pathway, tryptophan is metabolized through the serotonin pathway. In another, called the kynurenine pathway, tryptophan is used to make niacin (B3).The majority of dietary tryptophan (95%) is oxidized through the kynurenine pathway, and just a small portion is used for the synthesis of serotonin.

Indoleamine 2,3 dioxygenase (IDO) is one of the enzymes that degrades tryptophan in the kynurenine pathway. Tryptophan degradation by IDO is normally very moderate, but if tumor necrosis factor is elevated, IDO can be upregulated. The upregulation of IDO by tumor necrosis factor depletes tryptophan and creates an excess of toxic metabolites, such as kynurenine, kynurenic, and quinolinic acid.

The following study confirms kynurenine pathway (KYN-p) activity is involved in fibromyalgia and states that IDO enzyme inhibition may be a novel method for treating fibromyalgia fatigue.

STUDY

Kynurenine pathway activity linked to fibromyalgia fatigue.

Boomershine, C.S., D. Titova, C. Zhu, A.M. Oeser, M.W. Calcutt, A. Bian, T. Gebretsadik, R. Johnson, C. Michael Stein. 2009.

“Increased KYN-p activity is associated with FM fatigue in humans and a murine model. IDO enzyme inhibition may be a novel method for treating FM fatigue.”

The toxic metabolites produced through increased kynurenine pathway activity, kynurenine, kynurenic, and quinolinic acid, have been demonstrated to be involved in depression, bipolar disorder, low GABA, elevated glutamate, suicide, IBS, and inflammation of the fascia.

In our first study, researchers discuss the major role that the potentially neurotoxic kynurenine metabolites, kynurenine and quinolinic acid, play in depression. They also state that the depression in inflammation-associated depression is a “late” phenomenon that develops over a background of sickness. In other words, you aren’t physically sick because you are depressed; it is the other way around.

In addition, the study authors state that research has revealed that alterations in brain serotonin levels *do not* play a major role in depression, especially when compared to activation of the kynurenine pathway.

STUDY

Inflammation-associated depression: from serotonin to kynurenine.

Dantzer, R., J.C. O'Connor, M.A. Lawson, K.W. Kelley. 2011. *Psychoneuroendocrinology* 36(3):426-36. Epub 2010 Oct 30.

"In the field of depression, inflammation-associated depression stands up as an exception since its causal factors are obvious and it is easy to mimic in an animal model...These clinical studies have revealed that depression is a late phenomenon that develops over a background of early appearing sickness. Incorporation of this feature in animal models of inflammation-associated depression has allowed the demonstration that alterations of brain serotoninergic neurotransmission do not play a major role in the pathogenesis. This is in contrast to the activation of the tryptophan degrading enzyme indoleamine 2,3-dioxygenase that generates potentially neurotoxic kynurenine metabolites such as 3-hydroxy kynurenine and quinolinic acid."

In the following study from the Karolinska Institute in Stockholm, Sweden, the institute that awards the Nobel prizes in medicine, researchers found elevated brain levels of kynurenic acid (KYNA) in bipolar disorder.

STUDY

Elevated levels of kynurenic acid in the cerebrospinal fluid of patients with bipolar disorder.

Olsson, S.K., M. Samuelsson, P. Saetre, L. Lindström, E.G. Jönsson, C. Nordin, G. Engberg, S. Erhardt, M. Landén. 2010. *J Psychiatry Neurosci.* 35(3):195-9.

"Brain KYNA levels are increased in euthymic men with bipolar disorder. These findings indicate shared mechanisms between bipolar disorder and schizophrenia. Elevated levels of brain KYNA may provide further insight to the pathophysiology and progression of bipolar disorder."

In the following study, researchers found that kynurenine was able to induce convulsions by displacing GABA. The researchers concluded, "The data suggest that the convulsant activity of L-kynurenine might be due to interaction with GABA receptors."

STUDY

Kynurenine may directly interact with GABA receptors in rat brain.

Pinelli, A., S. Govoni, C. Ossi, F. Battaini, B.R. Caimi, S. Trivulzio. 1985. *Pharmacology* 30(5):255-8.

"Previous studies have shown that kynurenine may have convulsant activity...kynurenine was able to displace 3H-GABA from rat brain membrane preparations. The data suggest that the convulsant activity of L-kynurenine might be due to an interaction with GABA receptors..."

In our next study researchers found that quinolinic acid reduced GABA in a dose-dependent manner.

STUDY

Modulation of striatal quinolinate neurotoxicity by elevation of endogenous brain kynurenic acid.

Harris, C.A., A.F. Miranda, J.J. Tanguay, R.J. Boegman, R.J. Beninger, K. Jhamandas. 1998. *Br J Pharmacol.* 124(2):391-9.

"Intrastriatal infusion of quinolinic acid also produced a dose-dependent reduction in striatal GABA content."

Not only does quinolinic acid reduce GABA, but it increases glutamate, as the following study confirms.

STUDY

Quinolinic acid stimulates synaptosomal glutamate release and inhibits glutamate uptake into astrocytes.

Tavares, R.G., C.I. Tasca, C.E. Santos, L.B. Alves, L.O. Porciúncula, T. Emanuelli, D.O. Souza. 2002. *Neurochem Int.* 40(7):621-7.

"Quinolinic acid (QA) is an endogenous neurotoxin involved in various neurological diseases, whose action seems to be exerted via glutamatergic receptors... Enhanced synaptosomal glutamate release, associated with inhibition of glutamate uptake into astrocytes induced by QA could contribute to increase extracellular glutamate concentrations which ultimately lead to overstimulation of the glutamatergic system. These data provide additional evidence that neurotoxicity of QA may be also related to disturbances on the glutamatergic transport system, which could result in the neurological manifestations observed when this organic acid accumulates in the brain."

In the following study researchers concluded that kynurenine and related molecular pathways may be implicated in the pathophysiology of suicidal behavior.

STUDY

Plasma kynurenine levels are elevated in suicide attempters with major depressive disorder.

Sublette, M.E., H.C. Galfalyy, D. Fuchs, M. Lapidus, M.F. Grunebaum, M.A. Oquendo, J.J. Mann, T.T. Postolache. 2011. *Brain Behav Immun.* 25(6):1272-8.

“Inflammation has been linked to depression and suicide risk. One inflammatory process that has been minimally investigated in this regard is cytokine-stimulated production of kynurenine (KYN) from tryptophan (TRP). Recent data suggest that KYN increases in cerebrospinal fluid (CSF) are associated with depressive symptoms secondary to immune activation...These preliminary results suggest that KYN and related molecular pathways may be implicated in the pathophysiology of suicidal behavior.”

The following studies confirm that both males and females with irritable bowel syndrome (IBS) have abnormal tryptophan metabolism. Abnormal tryptophan metabolism is indeed the “common pathogenetic mechanism” that both fibromyalgia and IBS share. In addition, the researchers found that the higher the level of kynurenine, the more likely the patients were to suffer with anxiety and depression.

STUDY

Tryptophan catabolism in females with irritable bowel syndrome: relationship to interferon-gamma, severity of symptoms and psychiatric co-morbidity.

Fitzgerald, P., E.M. Cassidy, G. Clarke, P. Scully, S. Barry, E.M.M. Quigley, F. Shanahan, J. Cryan, T.G. Dinan. 2008. *Neurogastroenterol Motil.* 20(12):1291-7.

"Irritable bowel syndrome (IBS) has been linked with abnormal serotonin functioning and immune activation. Tryptophan forms the substrate for serotonin biosynthesis, but it can alternatively be catabolized to kynurenine (Kyn) by the enzyme indoleamine 2,3-dioxygenase (IDO)... Irritable bowel syndrome subjects had increased Kyn concentrations compared with controls...and there was a trend for Kyn:Trp to be increased in the IBS group... There was a positive correlation between IBS severity and Kyn:Trp... Those with severe IBS symptoms had increased Kyn:Trp compared to those with less severe symptoms and controls, and were over twice as likely to have depression or anxiety compared to those with less severe IBS... Females with IBS have abnormal Trp catabolism. The Kyn:Trp is related to symptom severity, and those with severe IBS symptoms have increased shunting of Trp along the Kyn pathway which contributes to the abnormal serotonergic functioning in this syndrome."

STUDY

Tryptophan degradation in irritable bowel syndrome: evidence of indoleamine 2,3-dioxygenase activation in a male cohort.

Clarke, G., P. Fitzgerald, J.F. Cryan, E.M. Cassidy, E.M. Quigley, T.G. Dinan. 2009. *BMC Gastroenterol.* 9:6.

"Both kynurenine levels and the kynurenine:tryptophan ratio were significantly increased in the IBS cohort compared with healthy controls...These findings suggest that the activity of IDO, the immunoresponsive enzyme which is responsible for the degradation of tryptophan along this pathway, is enhanced in IBS patients relative to controls."

Cartilage can also be affected by kynurenine. Patients with fibromyalgia often experience a condition known as costochondritis, which is an inflammation of the cartilage that connects a rib to the breastbone (sternum) -a junction known as the costosternal joint. In the following study researchers found that kynurenine inhibited chondrocyte (cartilage cell) proliferation in a dose-dependent manner, which led the researchers to conclude that kynurenine has a pathophysiological effect on cartilage in inflammatory arthropathies (joint diseases).

STUDY

Kynurenine inhibits chondrocyte proliferation and is increased in synovial fluid of patients with septic arthritis.

Lögters, T.T., M.D. Laryea, M. Jäger, M. Schädel-Höpfner, J. Windolf, S. Flohé, J. Altrichter, M. Scholz, A.N. Paunel-Görgülü. 2010. *J Orthop Res.* 28(11):1490-6.

"Kynurenine, the major degradation product of tryptophan has been shown to directly damage various tissues...Further, kynurenine inhibited chondrocyte (ATDC5) cell proliferation in a dose-dependent manner...Furthermore kynurenine inhibits proliferation of chondrocytes, which strongly suggests a pathophysiological effect of kynurenine on cartilage in inflammatory arthropathies."

In the following study researchers identified kynurenine as a blood marker for interstitial cystitis (IC) in both humans and cats with feline IC. Interstitial Cystitis, also known as painful bladder syndrome, is a chronic, oftentimes painful, inflammatory condition of the bladder that often affects fibromyalgia patients. The researchers collected samples from humans with IC, healthy humans, and humans with other urological illnesses. They also collected samples from cats with feline IC, healthy cats, and cats with other diseases. They discovered similar increased levels of kynurenine (at least 20 percent more) in both the human IC blood samples and feline IC blood samples, but not in the other samples.

STUDY

A candidate serum biomarker for bladder pain syndrome/interstitial cystitis.

Rubio-Diaz, D.E., M.E. Pozza, J. Dimitrakov, J.P. Gilleran, M.M. Giusti, J.L. Stella, L.E. Rodriguez-Saona, C.A. Buffington. 2009. *Analyst* 134(6):1133-7. Epub 2009 Apr 16.

"Analysis of cat samples using liquid chromatography-mass spectroscopy revealed differences in the concentration of tryptophan and its metabolites between healthy and affected cats. These results demonstrate the potential utility of infrared microspectroscopy to diagnose IC in both humans and cats."

It is not surprising that tryptophan metabolites are linked to interstitial cystitis. In the following study, the researchers state that these metabolites produced bladder cancer when implanted in the bladder.

STUDY

Possible roles of excess tryptophan metabolites in cancer.

Chung, K.T., G.S. Gadupudi. 2011. *Environ Mol Mutagen.* 52(2):81-104. doi: 10.1002/em.20588.

"These metabolites could interact with nitrite to become mutagenic nitrosamines. They could be a promoter in the initiator-promoter model of carcinogenesis. They produced bladder cancer when implanted in the bladder."

Kynurenine pathway activity is also linked to damaged fascia. In the following study, the researchers found that the toxic tryptophan metabolites, kynurenine and quinolinic acid, led to the fascia becoming "inflamed and fibrotic."

STUDY

Scleroderma, fasciitis, and eosinophilia associated with the ingestion of tryptophan.

Silver, R.M., M.P. Heyes, J.C. Maize, B. Quearry, M. Vionnet-Fuasset. 1990. *N Engl J Med.* 322:874-881.

"The fascia was inflamed and fibrotic...Plasma levels of L-kynurenine and quinolinic acid, which are metabolites of tryptophan, were significantly higher- findings consistent with the activation of the enzyme indoleamine-2,3-dioxygenase."

Since the body is producing toxic tryptophan metabolites in fibromyalgia, it would be unwise to take additional tryptophan in supplement form. In addition to fasciitis, tryptophan supplements such as 5-Hydroxytryptophan (5-HTP), have been linked to scleroderma, blood abnormalities (eosinophilia), and eosinophilia-myalgia syndrome, a serious condition involving extreme muscle tenderness (Silver, 1990).

CHAPTER 9

Scientific Findings:

Low Growth Hormone Secretion, Low Somatomedin C, and Low Levels of Endorphins

OUR NEXT FINDINGS ARE low growth hormone secretion, low somatomedin C, and low levels of endorphins.

LOW GROWTH HORMONE SECRETION

The researchers from the following study found that patients with fibromyalgia had a significantly *lower secretion of growth hormone.*

STUDY

Low growth hormone secretion in patients with fibromyalgia--a preliminary report on 10 patients and 10 controls.

Bagge, E., B.A. Bengtsson, L. Carlsson, J. Carlsson. 1998. *J Rheumatol.* 25(1):145-8.

"A significantly lower secretion of growth hormone was found in the patients in comparison with healthy controls."

Growth hormone (GH), or somatropin, is the most abundant hormone produced by the pituitary gland and the body's foremost anti-ageing hormone. Growth hormone stimulates growth, cell reproduction, and regeneration. It is essential for normal muscle metabolism and repair. Growth hormone also regulates the amount of sugar in the blood and promotes the breakdown of fat.

Many people believe that as we age the amount of GH in our body decreases. In fact, the difference, generally, in growth hormone levels between adults and adolescents is not in the amount of GH, but in its release. For instance, adequate amounts of blood protein levels will stimulate the release of GH from the pituitary gland. The inability to digest proteins, due to a lack of protease, would result not only in a reduction of the amount of GH, but also a reduction in the release of GH from the pituitary. In the following study researchers concluded that dietary protein restriction not only reduced the amount of GH, it also blunted the release of GH from the pituitary.

STUDY

Dietary protein restriction impairs both spontaneous and growth hormone-releasing factor-stimulated growth hormone release in the rat.

Harel, Z. and G.S. Tannenbaum. 1993. *Endocrinology* 133(3):1035-43.

"These results demonstrate that lack of dietary protein blunts spontaneous pulsatile GH release...and reduces pituitary GH content and size."

LOW SOMATOMEDIN C

Patients with fibromyalgia also have significantly lower levels of a by-product of growth hormone (GH) called *somatomedin C*, as the following study confirms. The researchers measured somatomedin C because GH has a very short half-life. In addition, the researchers state that somatomedin C is the major mediator of GH's anabolic actions and is a prerequisite for normal muscle homeostasis.

STUDY

Low levels of somatomedin C in patients with the fibromyalgia syndrome. A possible link between sleep and muscle pain.

Bennett, R.M., S.R. Clark, S.M. Campbell, C.S. Burckhardt. 1992. *Arthritis Rheum.* 35(10):1113-6.

"Because growth hormone has a very short half-life, serum levels of somatomedin C were measured; somatomedin C is the major mediator of growth hormone's anabolic actions and is a prerequisite for normal muscle homeostasis...Significantly lower levels of somatomedin C were observed in the fibromyalgia patients compared with controls... These findings indicate that there is a distinctive disruption of the growth hormone-somatomedin C neuroendocrine axis in a majority of fibromyalgia patients."

In the following study the researchers concluded that protein intake was a regulator of somatomedin-C in adult humans.

STUDY

Dietary components that regulate serum somatomedin-C concentrations in humans.

Isley, W.L., L.E. Underwood, D.R. Clemmons. 1983. *J Clin Invest.* 71(2): 175–182.

"We conclude that both protein and energy intake are regulators of serum somatomedin-C concentrations in adult humans... The correlation between changes in somatomedin-C and nitrogen balance

> suggests that the former are directly related to changes in protein synthesis and may be helpful in assessing the response to nutritional therapy."

SYMPTOMS OF LOW ADULT GROWTH HORMONE

- A higher level of body fat, especially around the waist
- Anxiety and depression
- Changes in the makeup of the blood cholesterol. People with adult growth hormone deficiency have higher than normal levels of low-density lipoproteins in comparison to their high density lipoproteins. They also tend to have higher triglyceride levels. (Triglycerides are another type of fat that circulates in the blood and contributes to blocked blood vessels.)
- Decreased sexual function and interest
- Fatigue
- Feelings of being isolated from other people
- Greater sensitivity to heat and cold
- Less muscle (lean body mass)
- Less strength, stamina and ability to exercise without taking a rest
- Reduced bone density and a tendency to have more bone fractures as they get older (Cedars Sinai, 2012).

Low Endorphins

Fibromyalgia patients also have *lower levels of endorphins*. Endorphin is a term used to identify a group of naturally-occurring compounds that act as the body's painkillers. Primary among them are the beta-endorphins and the enkephalins. The following study found that fibromyalgia patients had significantly lower levels of beta-endorphins.

STUDY

Peripheral blood mononuclear cell beta-endorphin concentration is decreased in chronic fatigue syndrome and fibromyalgia but not in depression: preliminary report.

Panerai, A.E., J. Vecchiet, P. Panzeri, P. Meroni, S. Scarone, E. Pizzigallo, M.A. Giamberardino, P. Sacerdote. 2002. *Clin J Pain.* 18(4):270-3.

"Beta-endorphin concentrations were significantly lower in patients with chronic fatigue syndrome or fibromyalgia syndrome than in normal subjects..."

Endorphins are morphine-like substances that block pain signals in the spinal cord and brain stem. They do this by binding to the same receptor sites that pain signals use.

The body's goal in pain suppression is to allow the body to cope with pain while remaining focused, rather than allowing the perception of pain to overwhelm the system and cause panic and confusion. Endorphins are released by the brain and central nervous system when the brain perceives pain. They dull the sensation of pain and also help the individual cope with the emotional aspects of pain by changing the way the pain is perceived. Since endorphins can influence perception, they also play a role in memory formation and mood, helping people feel joy, contentment, and general well-being.

Beta-endorphins are peptides-small proteins that consist of short chains of amino acids. Therefore, amino acids are needed to produce beta-endorphins. Specific amino acids needed to produce the beta-endorphin peptide are: phenylalanine, tyrosine, threonine, valine, leucine, and methionine. We have shown that these specific amino acids are found lacking in patients with fibromyalgia (Bazzichi, 2009).

One of the drugs often used to treat fibromyalgia is the opiate antagonist low dose naltrexone (LDN). It was initially approved by the FDA to treat heroin addiction. Low doses of naltrexone are thought to work by temporarily blocking the body's ability to release endorphins by binding to the same receptor sites. The body compensates by producing more endorphins than it typically would once the drug wears off. If you lack the ability to make endorphins though, this accelerated response could just could just further deplete your body's long term ability to produce endorphins.

CHAPTER 10

Scientific Findings:

Comorbidity with Rheumatoid Arthritis, Osteoporosis, Low Calcium, and Low Vitamin D

Our next findings are *comorbidity with rheumatoid arthritis*, osteoporosis, low calcium, and low vitamin D.

Comorbidity With Rheumatoid Arthritis

There is an association between fibromyalgia and rheumatoid arthritis. "Arthritis Today states, "About 20 to 30 percent of people with rheumatoid arthritis also develop fibromyalgia, although no one knows why" (Arthritis Today, 2009).

Fibromyalgia and rheumatoid arthritis (RA) are both associated with osteoporosis, low calcium, and low vitamin D.

Osteoporosis

The following study published in the *Journal of Rheumatology* shows the increased risk fibromyalgia patients have for developing osteoporosis. The study concludes that fibromyalgia (FM) was frequently associated with osteoporosis.

STUDY

Fibromyalgia: a risk factor for osteoporosis.

Swezey, R.L., J. Adams. 1999. *J Rheumatol* 26(12):2642-4.

"FM in this pilot study was frequently associated with osteoporosis."

LOW CALCIUM

Fibromyalgia patients also have low calcium. The following study found that fibromyalgia patients had significantly *reduced intracellular calcium.*

STUDY

Role of intracellular calcium ions in the physio-pathology of fibromyalgia syndrome.

Magaldi, M., L. Moltoni, G. Biasi, R. Marcolongo. 2000. *Boll Soc Ital Biol Sper.* 76(1-2):1-4.

"The results obtained show that in fibromyalgia patients the intra-cellular calcium concentration is significantly reduced in comparison to that of healthy controls..."

In addition, the following hair analysis study found that fibromyalgia patients had "significantly higher calcium and magnesium levels than the control subjects." In order to understand the results of this study, it is important to note that when a hair analysis finds a high amount of calcium, it usually indicates a deficiency of calcium in the body. The high calcium reading often represents a loss of calcium into the *soft tissues*. One reason for the loss is that the calcium consumed was not able to be assimilated.

STUDY

Hair calcium and magnesium levels in patients with fibromyalgia: a case center study.

Sy, Ng. 1999. *J Manipulative Physiol Ther.* 22(9):586-93.

"Wilcoxon rank sum tests showed that patients with fibromyalgia had significantly higher calcium and magnesium levels than the control subjects..."

LOW VITAMIN D

Vitamin D deficiency is also common in fibromyalgia, as the following study states.

STUDY

Vitamin D deficiency is associated with anxiety and depression in fibromyalgia.

Armstrong, D.J., G.K. Meenagh, I. Bickle, A.S. Lee, E.S. Curran, M.B. Finch. 2007. *Clin Rheumatol.* (4):551-4.

"Vitamin D deficiency is common in fibromyalgia and occurs more frequently in patients with anxiety and depression. The nature and direction of the causal relationship remains unclear, but there are definite implications for long-term bone health."

Notice the study points out the implications of a vitamin D deficiency for long-term bone health. The inability to digest proteins, due to a lack of protease, would prevent your body from properly metabolizing calcium and vitamin D, which could then lead to osteoporosis and arthritis.

Lita Lee, Ph.D., a chemist and enzyme nutritionist, explained the connection well when she wrote:

> "All forms of arthritis involve abnormal calcium metabolism. Ninety-nine percent of the body calcium is (or should be) in the bones and teeth. The other one percent, found in the blood, is just as important because it is essential in the blood clotting mechanism, muscle and nerve function, vitamin D function, and the function of hormones that control calcium metabolism (called parathyroid hormones). Of the one percent of calcium in the blood, half is protein-bound and half is ionized. Both require adequate protein digestion. If you are deficient in protein because you can't digest it, you cannot carry protein-bound calcium. If you lack optimum acidity from inadequate digestion of protein, you will not have enough ionized calcium. In either case, you are a candidate for arthritis.
>
> The abnormal deposit of calcium is one of the factors involved in arthritis and arthritic inflammation. Soft tissue, any kind of body tissue other than bones and teeth, is a target for depositing calcium. Wherever this happens, pathology occurs: in the joints, around inflamed areas (osteoarthritis), in the arteries (arteriosclerosis), in the kidneys (kidney stones), in the soft lenses of the eyes (cataracts), in the brain (stroke) and so on" (Lee, 2009).

The inability to carry protein-bound calcium would explain the low levels of vitamin D and calcium found in fibromyalgia and RA. Without blood-borne calcium, you would not be able to properly metabolize vitamin D. As Dr. Lee stated, blood-borne calcium is essential for vitamin D function. The problem lies in the *binding and transport*, just as with vitamin B12.Taking additional vitamin D or calcium in supplement form, that you are not able to properly metabolize, would just give your body more vitamin D and calcium to deposit in your joints and soft tissue (such as was found in the fibromyalgia hair analysis study).

It may also lead to another disease called sarcoidosis. Sarcoidosis is an inflammatory condition that produces tiny lumps of cells called granulomas in various organs of the body. These granulomas clump together into large or small groups, resulting in organ damage. Dysregulated calcium and vitamin D metabolism are well-recognized features of sarcoidosis.

The inability to properly metabolize vitamin D and calcium can also affect the muscles. Muscle weakness, pain, muscle cramps and twitching are all associated with vitamin D and calcium deficiency.

Vitamin D plays a role in regulating cellular processes in the nervous system and muscle tissue. Without proper levels of vitamin D, electrical impulses along nerve pathways may begin to misfire, causing muscles at different locations in the body to contract and relax.

Low calcium can cause nerve cells to become extra sensitive to sodium and fire too often, causing muscle cramping and pain. Calcium is also found inside the muscle in a sort of pocket called the sarcoplasmic reticulum (SR).When the nerves send a signal for the muscles to contract, the SR releases calcium. The calcium then binds to a protein within the muscle fiber causing it to change shape and initiating a chain reaction that causes the muscle to contract. If there is not enough calcium in the SR, the muscle will fail to contract properly.

Proper muscle function can be restored, without the risk of additional disease symptoms, by restoring your body's ability to carry protein-bound calcium.

The inability to carry protein-bound calcium could also lead to osteoporosis. When the blood cannot carry protein-bound calcium because it lacks protein, it withdraws the necessary calcium from the bones to maintain homeostasis or internal balance. The bones need sufficient calcium to develop and maintain bone structure.

A lack of vitamin D would also play a role in osteoporosis. Vitamin D helps the bones absorb calcium and hold onto minerals. The higher a bone's mineral content, the stronger it is.

As we would expect, osteoporosis is also a common feature in patients with RA. In a 2006 British study, it was found that people with RA are 50% more likely to develop osteoporosis (van Staa, 2006). The study, of approximately 30,000 people with RA, found that the risk of osteoporosis existed even if no other risk factor, such as the long-term use of corticosteroids or smoking, was present. In fact, the risk posed by RA alone, was as great as the risk caused by taking corticosteroids.

CHAPTER 11

Scientific Findings:

Low Zinc, Low Stomach Acid, Small Intestine Bacterial Overgrowth (SIBO), and Increased Intestinal Permeability

OUR NEXT FINDINGS ARE low zinc, low stomach acid, small intestine bacterial overgrowth (SIBO), and increased intestinal permeability.

LOW ZINC

The following study found that patients with fibromyalgia (FM) have significantly *lower levels of zinc.*

STUDY

The relationship between serum trace element levels and clinical parameters in patients with fibromyalgia.

Sendur, O.F., E. Tastaban, Y. Turan, C. Ulman. 2008. *Rheumatol Int.* 28(11):1117-21.

"Serum levels of zinc... were significantly decreased by FM groups... According to the results of this study, it was asserted that... zinc levels may play an important role in the pathophysiology of FM."

According to the National Institutes of Health Office for Dietary Supplements, the main source for zinc is animal-based protein foods, such as poultry, red meat, oysters, eggs, seafood, and milk (National Institutes of Health, 2011). The inability to break down these foods would account for the low levels of zinc found in fibromyalgia.

Zinc is involved in a wide range of functions that are essential for both physical and mental health. The body needs zinc to make proteins and DNA, the genetic material in all cells. Zinc also helps wounds heal and is important for proper senses of taste and smell.

Zinc is an important mineral for the proper functioning of the immune system. According to the Office of Dietary Supplements, even a moderate deficiency of zinc can negatively affect natural killer cell activity and white blood cell functions.

Zinc is also required for the catalytic activity of approximately 300 enzymes. One of these enzymes is alcohol dehydrogenase, which is responsible for the detoxification of alcohol. The lack of zinc would explain the intolerance to alcohol that many patients with fibromyalgia experience.

In the following study the researchers found decreased alcohol dehydrogenase activity in zinc deficient (ZnD) rats, which resulted in a significant decrease in ethanol (alcohol) elimination.

STUDY

Effects of zinc deficiency on ethanol metabolism and alcohol and aldehyde dehydrogenase activities.

Das, I., R.E. Burch, H.K. Hahn. 1984. *J Lab Clin Med*. 104(4):610-7.

"There was a significant decrease in the ethanol elimination rate in rats given ZnD and ZnDE diets. Alcohol dehydrogenase activities in rats with deficient zinc levels also were decreased..."

Zinc is also necessary for carbonic anhydrase, the enzyme that makes stomach acid. Protease and stomach acid work in harmony to insure proper digestion of proteins, prevention of food allergies, vitamin B12 absorption, and to prevent an overgrowth of bacteria and yeast.

Low Stomach Acid

Dr. Sarah Myhill, M.D., a UK-based CFS/FM specialist, has found that *low stomach acid*, or hypochlorhydria, is especially common in those with fibromyalgia and chronic fatigue syndrome (Myhill, 2007). In speaking of the importance of sufficient stomach acid, Dr. Myhill states,

> "The stomach requires an acid environment for several reasons. First, acid is required for digestion of protein. Second, acid is required for the stomach to empty properly. Acid is also required to sterilize the stomach and kill bacteria and yeast that may be ingested.
>
> It is well known that the stomach must be acidic in order to absorb B12. Indeed, using a proton pump inhibitor such as Prilosec, often prescribed for patients with heartburn or GERD, will reduce absorption of B12 to less than 1% of expected. Many people already suffer from borderline B12 deficiency-this is a difficult vitamin for the body to assimilate, but essential for normal biochemistry. Hypochlorhydria can lead to allergies. The reason for this is that if foods are poorly digested then large antigenically interesting molecules get into the lower gut, where if the immune system reacts against them, that can switch on allergy."

One study found allergenic antigens were reduced up to 10,000-fold by adequate stomach acid (Untersmayr, 2006). People on acid-blocking medications were also 10.5 times more susceptible to IgE-mediated food reactions, with an elevation in IgE antibodies remaining five months after a three-month course of acid blocker therapy (Untersmayr, 2005).

Many people take acid-blocking medications in order to treat heartburn. If you frequently experience heartburn, you are not alone. The antacid industry generates 24 billion dollars a year (McCormick, 2005). The problem, however, isn't too much stomach acid, it's not enough. So, taking an antacid will actually make the problem worse.

Adequate production of stomach acid is required to close the muscular sphincter that relaxes and constricts to allow food to enter the stomach from the esophagus. When there is not enough stomach acid, the sphincter will not close, allowing what acid there is in the stomach to regurgitate into the esophagus.

SMALL INTESTINE BACTERIAL OVERGROWTH (SIBO)

Chronic fatigue syndrome (CFS) specialist Paul Cheney, M.D., has also found that most CFS and fibromyalgia patients have low stomach acid, which contributes to an overgrowth of bacteria in the small intestine (Sieverling, 2002). Dr. Cheney notes, "A UCLA study of 52 FM/CFS patients found *small intestine bacterial overgrowths (SIBO)* in ninety percent of the patients." In an additional study, published in *Annals of Rheumatic Diseases,* researchers found that *100%* (42/42) of the fibromyalgia patients tested had SIBO (Pimental, 2004).

In SIBO, the bacteria that overgrow are not necessarily pathogenic, but there are just too much of them in a section of the intestine where they shouldn't be in high numbers. Most of the bacteria in your intestines should actually be in your colon or large intestine, not in your small intestine. Small intestine bacterial overgrowth often manifests as bloating, gas, fatigue, and constipation.

Small intestine bacterial overgrowth can also develop if the pancreas lacks protease and other enzymes necessary for digestion. The pancreas normally secretes about a liter and a half of pancreatic enzymes into the duodenum every day for food digestion. Once food is broken down into easily usable fragments, it moves through the rest of the small intestine. A deficiency in digestive enzymes can lead to slow transit time and poorly absorbed food, which are ideal conditions for the development of SIBO.

Protease are also necessary for keeping the body free from parasites (such as intestinal worms), yeast overgrowth, and pathogenic bacteria and viruses. Parasites, fungal forms, and bacteria are *proteins* (protease digest proteins) that additionally disguise themselves in a protein shell that our bodies may view as normal. A virus is essentially a nucleic acid (DNA or RNA) enclosed in a protein shell.

Proteases work by removing this protein shell. With the protective barrier down, your immune system can then recognize and destroy the invading organism. Fibromyalgia patients often say their disease was preceded by a viral or bacterial infection. If you are bordering on a protease deficiency and you contract a viral or bacterial infection, this would further deplete your protease, as they would be needed to 'disarm' the invader.

An excess of pathogenic bacteria, yeast, and parasites can also lead to increased intestinal permeability or "leaky gut syndrome". Pathogenic yeasts, for instance, can grow into a fungal form with root-like tentacles that drill deep into the mucosal lining, poking "holes" in the gut. In addition, bacteria and yeasts give off toxins that can irritate the intestinal lining.

Increased intestinal permeability allows substances that would normally be blocked, such as toxins, microbes, undigested food, and waste to leak through the gut wall into the bloodstream. The immune system views these substances as foreign invaders, and rightly so. It starts making antibodies against the food particles, which leads to food allergies, and the constant stress put on the immune system to contain the toxins and microbes leads to inflammation and allergies throughout the body.

Increased Intestinal Permeability

Fibromyalgia patients have *increased intestinal permeability*, as the following study confirms.

STUDY

Altered intestinal permeability in patients with primary fibromyalgia and in patients with complex regional pain syndrome.

Goebel, A., S. Buhner, R. Schedel, H. Lochs, G. Sprotte. 2008. *Oxford Journals of Medicine Rheumatology* 47 (8): 1223-1227.

"The pain intensity of patients with FM has recently been reported to be correlated with the degree of small intestinal bacterial overgrowth (SIBO). SIBO is often associated with an increased intestinal permeability (IP). ...The IPs in primary FM and, unexpectedly, CRPS are increased. This study should stimulate further research to determine the implication of altered IP in the disease pathophysiology of FM and CRPS."

Zinc is also necessary for maintaining intestinal wall integrity. The following study found that zinc deficiency induced membrane barrier damage.

STUDY

Zinc deficiency induces membrane barrier damage and increases neutrophil transmigration in Caco-2 cells.

Finamore, A., M. Massimi, C.L. Devirgiliis, E. Megheri. 2008. *J Nutr.* 138(9):1664-70.

"These results provide new information on the critical role played by dietary zinc in the maintenance of membrane barrier integrity and in controlling inflammatory cell infiltration."

Even though zinc is an essential requirement for a healthy body, zinc, like iron, is a heavy metal ion and must be carefully controlled. Heavy metal ions are toxic to cells. Our bodies take great care to make sure metals go only where they need to and in exactly the right amount.

Scientists have discovered that metals, such as zinc, have special "chaperone" proteins that safely escort the metal through the interior of the cell and deliver it to the specific site where it is needed. Zinc also has "binding proteins" to prevent it from accumulating within the cell and poisoning the cell. The essential amino acid histidine is an essential component of zinc binding proteins, such as ZntR and Zur.

According to Thomas O'Halloran, professor of chemistry at Northwestern University, "The zinc regulatory system is so sensitive and finely tuned-at the femtomolar level-that the metal ions have no chance to float freely in the cell's cytoplasm before they are bound up in ZntR or Zur. Free floating zinc just doesn't exist" (Northwestern University, 2001).

Histidine was one of the essential amino acids found lacking in patients with fibromyalgia. Without histidine the body would not be able to properly bind zinc. We know that patients with fibromyalgia already lack one of the essential components to prevent zinc toxicity, but science doesn't fully understand the complexities involved in how the body protects itself from zinc while at the same time benefitting from it, so taking isolated zinc in supplement form could prove harmful.

CHAPTER 12

Scientific Findings:

Multiple Chemical Sensitivity, Low Cortisol, Low Estrogen, Low DHEA, and Low Testosterone

---

OUR NEXT FINDINGS ARE multiple chemical sensitivity, low cortisol, low estrogen, low DHEA, and low testosterone.

MULTIPLE CHEMICAL SENSITIVITY

The following study found that more than half of the fibromyalgia (FM) patients tested met the criteria for *multiple chemical sensitivity (MCS).*

STUDY

The relationship between fibromyalgia and the multiple chemical sensitivity syndrome.

Slotkoff, A. T., D. A. Radulovic, D. J. Clauw. 1997. *Annals of Internal Medicine* Vol. 26, No. 5 , Pages 364-367.

"Thirty-three of 60 patients with FM met the criteria for MCS. Eleven of these patients also fulfilled more restrictive criteria, requiring a "higher degree" of chemical sensitivity. MCS may represent an additional symptom complex within the spectrum of FM."

LOW CORTISOL AND LOW ESTROGEN

In the following study researchers found that fibromyalgia patients had significantly *lower levels of cortisol*. The researchers also discuss additional study findings that confirm *lower levels of estrogen* in patients with fibromyalgia.

STUDY

Cortisol and hypothalamic–pituitary–gonadal axis hormones in follicular-phase women with fibromyalgia and chronic fatigue syndrome and effect of depressive symptoms on these hormones.

Gur, Ali, R. Cevik, K. Nas, L. Colpan, S. Sarac. Published online 2004 March 15.

"Cortisol levels were significantly lower in patients with fibromyalgia or CFS than in healthy controls...Riedel and colleagues investigated female fibromyalgia patients and controls who were all in the follicular phase of their menstrual cycle. They found that fibromyalgia patients had significantly lower estrogen levels despite elevated FSH levels (Riedel, 1998)."

SYMPTOMS OF LOW CORTISOL

- Fatigue
- Poor response and "crashing" during stress
- Achiness
- Hypoglycemia (low blood sugar with irritability when hungry)
- Low blood pressure

SYMPTOMS OF LOW ESTROGEN	
• Fatigue	• Hot flashes
• Forgetfulness	• Night sweats
• Insomnia	• Depression
• Lack of sexual desire	• Irritability
• Painful intercourse	• Osteoporosis
• Early menopause	• Inability to become pregnant

Low DHEA and Low Testosterone

In our next study researchers found that fibromyalgia patients had significantly *reduced levels of DHEA*. Premenopausal fibromyalgia patients also had significantly *decreased testosterone (T) levels*.

STUDY

Hyposecretion of adrenal androgens and the relation of serum adrenal steroids, serotonin and insulin-like growth factor-1 to clinical features in women with fibromyalgia.

Dessein, P.H., E. A. Shipton, B.I. Joffe, D.P. Hadebe, A.E. Stanwix, B.A. Van der Merwe. 1999. *Pain* 83(2):313-9.

"DHEAS levels were decreased significantly in pre- and postmenopausal patients and T levels were decreased significantly in premenopausal...patients."

SYMPTOMS OF LOW DHEA	
• Fatigue	• Decreased stamina and alertness
• Depression	• Less muscle and bone mass
• Aching joints	• Low libido
• Dry skin and eyes	• Poor memory
• Weight gain	

SYMPTOMS OF LOW TESTOSTERONE IN MEN

- Infertility
- Decreased sexual function and desire
- Erectile dysfunction (ED)
- Hair loss
- Decreased muscle mass
- Osteoporosis

SYMPTOMS OF LOW TESTOSTERONE IN WOMEN

- Hot flashes
- Irritability
- Loss of sexual desire
- Sleep disturbances
- Loss of muscle mass
- Decreased bone density (osteoporosis)

Chemical sensitivity and the low hormone levels found in patients with fibromyalgia can be clearly explained by a disruption in the cytochrome P450 enzyme system.

Our bodies' first line of defense against chemicals and environmental pollutants is a powerful enzyme detoxification system called cytochrome P450. The cytochrome P450 system detoxifies all sorts of different chemicals that we eat and breathe, including drugs, carcinogens formed in cooking, and poisonous compounds in plants (Guengerich, 2008). For instance, cytochrome P450 is the reason doctors tell you not to drink grapefruit juice when taking certain medications. Grapefruits contain a flavinol molecule that inhibits cytochrome P450 enzymes. This would slow down the detoxification of the drug and might cause it to have a stronger effect than intended.

A disruption in the cytochrome P450 enzyme system would account for the chemical sensitivity found in patients with fibromyalgia. The lack of iron and B12 found in patients with fibromyalgia would lead to a disruption in the cytochrome P450 enzyme system.

The active site of cytochrome P450 contains a *heme iron* center, and therefore, cytochrome P450 enzymes are *hemoproteins*. Heme is made up of a squarish molecule--called a porphyrin--with an iron atom in the center. A molecule of iron is needed to make heme.

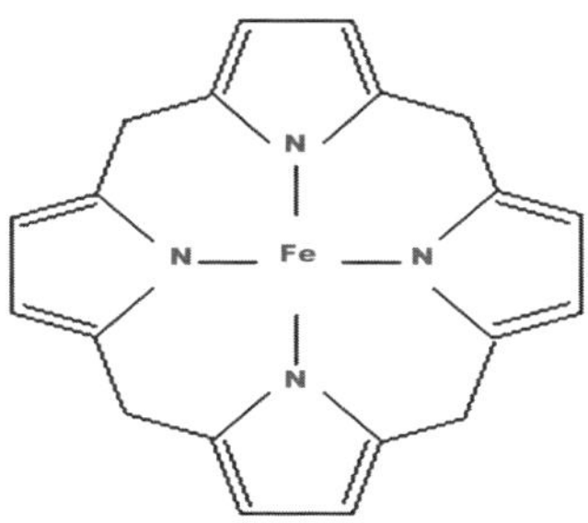

Figure 5. Heme Molecule

Vitamin B12 is also essential in the production of heme. The body makes heme mostly in the bone marrow and liver. The process of making heme is called the heme biosynthetic pathway. Each step of the process is controlled by one of eight enzymes. If any one of the eight enzymes is deficient, the pathway is disrupted.

The first component in the heme pathway is succinyl-CoA. Vitamin B12 serves as a cofactor for methylmalonyl-CoA mutase which converts methylmalonyl-CoA to succinyl-CoA. Therefore, a vitamin B12 deficiency would lead to a failure in the entire heme pathway.

The cytochrome P450 enzyme system also plays an essential role in hormone synthesis. It converts cholesterol into pregnenolone, which then gets converted into other hormones like estrogen, testosterone, cortisol, and DHEA. An inability to properly metabolize hormones, due to a disruption in the cytochrome P450 enzyme system, would account for the low hormone levels found in patients with fibromyalgia.

CHAPTER 13

Scientific Finding:
Comorbidity with Lupus

Our next finding is *comorbidity with lupus.*

Comorbidity with Lupus

The Lupus Foundation of America states, "Fibromyalgia affects about 30 percent of people with lupus" (Lupus Foundation of America, 2011).

It is not surprising that there is an association between lupus and fibromyalgia. Protease work alongside another digestive enzyme called deoxyribonuclease or DNase 1. Protease digest the proteins in the foods we eat and DNase 1 digests the DNA. The lack of DNase 1 has been determined to be a *causative* factor of lupus in numerous studies. As the following studies show, when this enzyme is removed in mice, the mice get lupus. When it is genetically modified in humans, lupus is the result.

STUDY

Lupus and deoxyribonuclease.

Lachmann, P.J., 2003. *Lupus* 12(3):202-6.

"Mice whose DNase 1 gene is knocked out are known to develop lupus and to be otherwise normal."

STUDY

Mutation of DNASE 1 in people with systemic lupus erythematosus.

Yasutomo, K., T. Horiuchi, S. Kagami, H. Tsukamoto, C. Hashimura, M. Urushihara, Y. Kuroda. 2001. Nat. Genet. 28(4):313-4.

“These data are consistent with the hypothesis that a direct connection exists between low activity of DNASE 1 and progression of human SLE.”

CHAPTER 14

Spinal Fluid Studies—These Don't Lie

NEXT, WE WOULD LIKE TO DISCUSS the results of some of the most definitive scientific findings to date in fibromyalgia and chronic fatigue syndrome. We are talking about spinal fluid studies.

CEREBROSPINAL FLUID ABNORMAL PROTEINS

In the following spinal fluid study from Georgetown University, researchers examined the cerebrospinal fluid of two independent cohorts of patients with overlapping fibromyalgia, chronic fatigue syndrome (CFS), and Persian Gulf War illness and discovered an *identical* set of *abnormal proteins*. The researchers stated, "This pilot study detected an identical set of central nervous system, innate immune and amyloidogenic proteins in cerebrospinal fluids from two independent cohorts of subjects with overlapping CFS, PGI (Persian Gulf War Illness), and fibromyalgia. Although syndrome names and definitions were different, the proteome and presumed pathological mechanisms may be shared." In other words, these diseases may be one and the same.

STUDY

A chronic fatigue syndrome – related proteome in human cerebrospinal fluid

Baraniuk, J.N., B. Casado, H. Maibach, D.J. Clauw, L.K. Pannell, S. Hess. 2005. BMC Neurol. 5:22.

"This pilot study detected an identical set of central nervous system, innate immune and amyloidogenic proteins in cerebrospinal fluids from two independent cohorts of subjects with overlapping CFS, PGI (Persian Gulf War Illness), and fibromyalgia. Although syndrome names and definitions were different, the proteome and presumed pathological mechanisms may be shared."

On Feb. 23, 2011, the Wall Street Journal reported on the results of another CFS spinal fluid study completed at the University of Medicine and Dentistry of New Jersey – New Jersey Medical School that also identified abnormal proteins specific to CFS that were not found in post-treatment lyme disease patients. In response to these findings, Suzanne Vernon, the scientific director of the Chronic Fatigue and Immune Dysfunction Syndrome Association of America stated, "They looked at a really important fluid, using a really advanced technology and they found clear differences. I'm very excited about this-you can't dispute these biological findings" (Schutzer, 2011).

A recent follow-up spinal fluid study from Georgetown University revealed more information about the source of the abnormal proteins found in fibromyalgia, CFS, and PGI (Johnson, 2010).

These abnormal proteins consisted of the following:

- Two proteins suggesting a protease–antiprotease imbalance is present.

- Several proteins suggesting small amounts of bleeding in the brain could be caused by the aggregation of proteins (amyloids) in the blood vessel.
- An additional protein suggests increased free radical production is present.
- Another protein is associated with inflammation.
- Another suggests problems with the vasoconstriction of the blood vessels and damage to the cells lining the blood vessels (the endothelial cells).
- An alternate protein suggesting altered rates of cell suicide (apoptosis) is present.

We can account for each and every one of these protein findings.

It should come as no surprise that the first protein finding reveals the direct involvement of protease in the disease process of fibromyalgia (and in CFS and PGI as well).

Amyloid proteins are revealed in the second finding and appear to be key elements of the protein signature. A lack of protease would lead to the formation of amyloid proteins. Amyloid proteins are peptides (short chains of amino acids) that get folded improperly as they are being made. Proteins trigger cellular activity by locking into each other like three dimensional keys. Since shape in a protein is everything, improper folding can cause a protein to be useless or even dangerous. It is the amino acid sequence of a protein that determines its specific shape and function. As we have shown, fibromyalgia patients lack numerous essential amino acids. These amino acids would be necessary for the formation of normal bodily proteins.

The final protein findings; increased free radical production, inflammation, problems with the vasoconstriction of the blood vessels, damage to the cells lining the blood vessels (the endothelial cells), and altered rates of cell suicide (apoptosis) would all be directly linked to the elevated levels of homocysteine found in patients with fibromyalgia.

CHAPTER 15

Vitamin B12– Is It Really Normal?

WE OFTEN HEAR, "I've had my B12 levels checked. They are normal." Let's take a closer look at the meaning of the word "normal". A study done at Tufts University may indicate that B12 deficiency is far more widespread than previously believed (McBride, 2000). The study looked at 3,000 individuals and found that 40% of the participants had low B12 values. Additionally, the study used 258 pg/mL as their criterion for a "low level." Other countries, however, use a much higher B12 level (approximately 500-600 pg/mL) to determine a deficiency. Of critical note; 500-600 pg/mL is the level at which memory loss, lethargy, and dementia can occur.

The levels of serum vitamin B12 considered normal in the United States are vastly lower than that of other countries like Japan and some European countries. American medical opinion defines blood levels lower than 200 pg/ mL as an indication of deficiency. This number is based on the level associated with the most severe manifestation of deficiency, which is pernicious anemia (abnormally formed red blood cells). Physicians in Japan and other countries consider blood levels of 500-1300 pg/mL to be the normal range. If you are within the "normal" range in the U.S., you have a severe deficiency-enough to cause pernicious anemia. Long before anemia becomes apparent, however, other symptoms manifest themselves. Symptoms such as muscle fatigue, shaking, burning sensations, pins and needles, irrational anger, memory loss, and impaired mental function may become evident. These neurological symptoms manifest themselves at approximately 500-600 pg/mL.

One surprising fact mentioned in the Tufts University study was that the participants were eating foods rich in vitamin B12, but their bodies were not absorbing the vitamin. As we have shown, the absorption of vitamin B12 is dependent on protease. No amount of vitamin B12 will reverse the symptoms of fibromyalgia associated with vitamin B12 deficiency, unless the mechanism your body has to absorb it is restored. The problem lies in the metabolism of B12, not just in the amount consumed. Proper absorption also depends on whether it is in natural or supplement form.

The absorption of vitamin B12 is an amazingly complex process. A recent study from Norway may be an indication that it might be best if we don't interfere with this process by taking vitamin B12 supplements.

In the study, published in the *Journal of the American Medical Association*, the researchers found that supplementation with vitamin B12 and folic acid increased the risk of being diagnosed with cancer, of dying from cancer, and of dying from any cause.

Here are the numbers:

"The study was a double-blind, placebo-controlled, randomized clinical trial in which nearly 7,000 adults in Norway were randomly selected to take one of the following:

- 0.8 mg of folic acid + 0.4 mg of vitamin B12 + 40 mg vitamin B6 per day
- 0.8 mg of folic acid + 0.4 mg of vitamin B12 per day
- 40 mg vitamin B6 per day
- placebo (no vitamins)

Double-blind means that neither the researchers nor the study participants knew who was taking which vitamins or the placebo. Randomized means that people were selected at random for each vitamin (or placebo) group. This type of study is considered "the gold standard" of research designs, because it is most likely to show results accurately, without errors that can happen with other study designs.

Study participants were followed for a median (similar to average) of approximately six and a half years (39 months of active study participation plus 38 months of post-study observation). The study showed that compared with people not receiving folic acid and vitamin B12, those who took these vitamins had:

- 21% higher risk of being diagnosed with cancer (any type)
- 38% higher risk of dying of cancer (any type)
- 18% higher risk of dying of any cause

Taking vitamin B6 did not have any measurable effects (good or bad) on the health of the study participants" (Dixon, 2009).

You may need to rethink everything you thought you knew about fighting your disease. You would not want to do anything that could possibly cause your body more harm. Your body can heal itself if it is given the raw materials it needs, in the form it was designed to use them in.

It is also important to avoid things that can deplete, block, or destroy vitamin B12.

Researchers from The National Institutes of Health warn us about the dangers of vitamin C supplements and the destruction of vitamin B12. They state, "Early research suggests that vitamin C supplements can destroy dietary vitamin B12" (National Institutes of Health, 2010).

Nitrous oxide anesthesia renders vitamin B12 inactive. Severe neurologic degeneration can result from the use of nitrous oxide in patients with a vitamin B12 deficiency. In the abstract entitled "Neurologic degeneration associated with nitrous oxide anesthesia in patients with vitamin B12 deficiency" the researchers state, "Patients with vitamin B12 deficiency are exceedingly sensitive to neurologic degeneration following nitrous oxide anesthesia" (Flippo, 1993).

Many people experience their first symptoms of fibromyalgia after a surgery and patients with existing fibromyalgia often find recovery from surgery can be slow and incomplete. The use of nitrous oxide during surgery may, in part, explain why.

Vaccinations containing thimerosal and other mercury-containing compounds should be avoided. Mercury can deplete vitamin B12 (Molecular Psychiatry, 2004).

Oral contraceptive use can also deplete vitamin B12. In the study entitled "Blood levels of homocysteine, folate, vitamin B6 and B12 in women using oral contraceptives compared to non-users" B12 levels were found to be "significantly lower" in oral contraceptive users than in non-users (Lussana, 2003). The subsequent rise in homocysteine, due to a lack of B12, would account for the increased risk of blood clots in women who use oral contraceptives.

Soy products contain vitamin B12 analogs (an inactive form our bodies can't use) and will actually increase the body's requirement for B12. In addition, trypsin (trypsin is a protease) inhibitors in soy interfere with protein digestion.

Smoking will deplete vitamin B12 and the heavy metals found in cigarette smoke can damage the pancreas (where protease originate). Cigarette smoke contains 4,000 chemical components, including over 30 heavy metals. Smoking has a recognized association with chronic pancreatitis and pancreatic cancer.

CHAPTER 16

Protease Supplements

THE PANCREAS RELEASES PROTEASE in an "inactive" form due to their strong potential to destroy the cells that produced them and to "digest" other parts of the body, such as the lining of the stomach. To protect the body's own cells inactive protease are secreted into the digestive tract and only activated when and where they are needed (Powell, 1999).

Research shows that supplementation with protease can destroy the body's lipases (Layer, 1993). These are the enzymes that digest fats. Supplemental protease can also lead to a serious condition involving damage to the large intestines called fibrosing colonopathy (Bakowski, 1999). In some cases, the problem was linked to the use of high supplemental amounts of enzymes (Milla, 1994). However, the amount of enzymes used has not been linked to the problem in all reports (Jones, 1995).

Our ultimate goal is to restore the health of the entire gastrointestinal (GI) tract in order to properly digest and metabolize proteins. As we have seen, the proper digestion and absorption of proteins requires the functional integrity of the entire gut. If the stomach lining or other parts of the GI tract are further damaged through the use of supplemental enzymes, then we will not be able to achieve our goal.

In addition, as serious a problem as the inability to digest proteins is, it would be equally as serious if the body were not able to digest fats. The destruction of the body's lipases by supplemental protease could lead to very harmful consequences.

CHAPTER 17

Women and Fibromyalgia

WOMEN ARE MORE PRONE to develop fibromyalgia. This could be due to differences in protein metabolism between men and women. Sex hormones play an important role in protein metabolism, as the following study confirms. Ovarian hormones inhibit protein synthesis, whereas testosterone increases protein synthesis.

STUDY

Gender differences in protein metabolism.

Tipton, K.D., 2001. Curr Opin Clin Nutr Metab Care. 4(6):493-8.

"Testosterone increases muscle protein synthesis and net muscle protein balance, resulting in increased muscle mass. Males and females have similar amounts of testosterone until puberty, then testosterone levels increase much more dramatically in males, as does muscle mass....In summary, differences in musculature point to differences in protein metabolism, especially muscle protein metabolism among males and females. It appears that sex hormones play an important role in any possible differences..."

Pregnancy and childbirth would also deplete vitamin B12. During pregnancy, extra red blood cells are needed for the mother and the developing fetus. Vitamin B12 is necessary for the formation of red blood cells.

The higher demand and ultimate depletion of vitamin B12 in pregnancy could also lead to an increased risk for fibromyalgia.

It is extremely important for a woman with fibromyalgia that becomes pregnant, or is thinking about becoming pregnant, to make sure she has adequate levels of vitamin B12. Low levels of vitamin B12 may increase the risk of neural tube defects, such as spina bifida. Neural tube defects refer to a group of birth defects that affect the brain and spinal cord.

A study conducted by researchers from the National Institute of Child Health and Human Development (NICHD) found that women with the lowest B12 levels had 5 times the risk of having a child with a neural tube defect compared to women with the highest B12 levels (Molloy, 2009). "Vitamin B12 is essential for the functioning of the nervous system and for the production of red blood cells," stated Duane Alexander, M.D., director of the NICHD. "The results of this study suggest that women with low levels of B12 not only may risk health problems of their own, but also may increase the chance that their children may be born with a serious birth defect."

CHAPTER 18

You Can Recover

THE FIRST DESCRIPTION OF FIBROMYALGIA in the medical literature was in 1843. It was described as a type of rheumatism "with painful hard places". The years since that time have been filled with debate over its actual existence. Fibromyalgia was finally accepted as a disease in just this last decade and granted an insurance number (CPT 729.1). Not much has changed in a century and a half; the physician still looks for painful hard places to make a diagnosis. The current method of diagnosis focuses on the finding of tenderness in at least 11 of 18 specific body points in the absence of any other disease.

Scientific research from around the world has shown that the disease process of fibromyalgia involves far more than what is currently being recognized. Now that you know why you are sick, we want you to be able to rely on this newfound knowledge to recover. You can recover by restoring your body's ability to digest proteins. You can recover by taking whole organic herbs to kill pathogenic yeasts and bacteria and to heal the intestinal wall. You can recover by avoiding things that destroy beneficial bacteria and enzymes. You can recover.

SECTION 2

THE CURE

CHAPTER 19

Food as Medicine

> *"The doctor of the future will give no medicine, but will interest her or his patients in the care of the human frame, in a proper diet, and in the cause and prevention of disease."*
> — *Thomas A. Edison, US inventor (1847–1931)*

In this portion of the book we will be discussing what Thomas Edison envisioned; using food as our medicine. Some foods can be extraordinarily healthy and beneficial, while others will only hinder your recovery. Simply because a food is marketed as "healthy" doesn't necessarily mean it is. Canola oil is one such food.

Canola Oil

One day, while preparing to make dinner, I went into my pantry to get some oil. I chose the canola oil I had recently purchased on a big city shopping trip to a Denver health food store. I didn't even make it through the pantry door. "Wait a minute," I thought, "what's a canola plant?" When I couldn't answer that question, I knew what I would be spending the rest of my day doing.

What I discovered made me realize that I had been on autopilot. We can't assume that just because something is marketed as healthy, that it truly is. So, what is a canola plant? Not something you would plant in your garden, I'm sure. Canola oil comes from the rapeseed plant. Rapeseed is the same plant that gave us mustard gas in WWI. It is toxic. Even the insects won't eat it. It is also cheap and plentiful. Canadian scientists figured out how to extract the chemical that would kill us immediately, and then began to market the remainder as a health food; hence the name, "canola oil", which is derived from "Canadian oil".

Producers of canola oil contribute five percent of their profits to the Canola Marketing Fund. I could go on and on about its structure and whether this oil, that can only be created in a laboratory, is something our bodies recognize. However, if it wasn't a food 100 years ago, it's not a food now. At least it shouldn't be.

There have also been various animal studies done, including one in Japan, during which the animals that ingested canola oil actually died (Dewey, 1997). Canola oil depletes the body of vitamin E, which is an essential antioxidant. The depletion of vitamin E results in increased dangerous free-radical activity. Free-radicals can cause widespread damage to your body.

Wonderful alternatives to canola oil include:

- Virgin coconut oil – for cooking at high temperatures, as it maintains its stability even at high heat. It is a healthful source of saturated fat in the form of medium chain triglycerides (MCTs). One of these MCTs is lauric acid, which supports the immune system.
- Extra virgin olive oil – for cooking at low temperatures or making a healthy salad dressing.
- Lard, tallow, and other animal fats from organic, grass-fed, pasture-raised animals – are a great source of conjugated linoleic acid (CLA) and vitamin D. Saturated fats help with maintaining hormone balance, brain function, and vitamin absorption.

- Organic grass-fed butter – is another great source of CLA, which has been shown in studies to help prevent cancer and help muscle building and fat burning.

"Just Eat the Box"

One of the biggest mistakes most of us make when we start to improve our diets is to continue to eat boxed cereal. We might switch from sugary cereals to an organic loop or whole grain puff. My sister did it. Her kitchen shelves are lined with different brands of organic boxed cereal. But are they really healthy? My sister thinks so. "There's nothing wrong with those," she says. "They're organic and whole grain." Is she right? I tell her she'd be better off just eating the box.

The reason is, nearly all packaged, dry cereals, even the organic ones, are produced by a process called extrusion. Sally Fallon, of the Weston A. Price Foundation, explains the process of extrusion:

> "Dry breakfast cereals are produced by a process called extrusion. Cereal makers first create a slurry (a thick suspension of solids in a liquid) of the grains and then put them in a machine called an extruder. The grains are then forced out of a little hole at high temperature and pressure. Depending on the shape of the hole, the grains are made into little O-shapes, flakes, animal shapes, or shreds (as in shredded wheat or TriscuitsR) or they are puffed (as in puffed rice). A blade slices off each little flake or shape, which is then passed by a nozzle and sprayed with a coating of oil and sugar to seal off the cereal from the ravages of milk and give it a crunch."

This process of 'extrusion' destroys many of the nutrients that are present in the grain and renders the amino acids toxic to our bodies by denaturing the proteins. The following two unpublished studies show just how harmful denatured proteins are to the human body:

In his book, *Fighting the Food Giants*, Paul Stitt cited a cereal company study in which four groups of rats were each given a different diet (Stitt, 1980).

1. The 1st group received plain whole wheat, water, vitamins and minerals.
2. The 2nd group received puffed wheat (an extruded cereal), water, vitamins and minerals.
3. The 3rd group received just water.
4. The 4th group received water, vitamins and minerals.

The rats that were part of the group that received the whole wheat (1st group) lived for over a year on the diet. The rats that received the water, vitamins and minerals (4th group) lived about two months. The rats that were only given water (3rd group) lived for a month. The most surprising results came from the group given the puffed wheat (2nd group). The rats that received the puffed wheat, water, vitamins and minerals lived for only about two weeks. Upon autopsy, researchers found signs of insulin shock, with dysfunction of the pancreas, liver, kidneys, and the degeneration of nerves of the spine.

In an additional study, University of Michigan researchers separated their rats into three groups (Fallon, 2008).

1. The 1st group received corn flakes and water.
2. The 2nd group received the cardboard box the cereal came in and water.
3. The 3rd group (the control group) received rat chow and water.

The control group remained in good health during the experiment. The rats fed the corn flake box and water died of malnutrition. The rats given the corn flakes and water, however, died before the rats that just ate the box! Additionally, the rats given the corn flakes displayed schizophrenic behavior before they died; throwing fits, biting each other, and finally going into convulsions. See why I told my sister she'd be better off eating the box?

TRANS FATS AND CANDLE WAX. IT'S WHAT'S FOR DINNER.

When William Procter and James Gamble started their company, Procter & Gamble®, they hired a chemist, E.C. Kayster, to develop a process to hydrogenate cottonseed oil. This process would ensure the shortening would remain solid at normal storage temperatures. This was in 1911. The initial purpose was to create a cheaper substance to make candles, rather than the expensive animal fats which were in use at the time.

Electricity began to diminish the candle market, and since the product looked like lard they began selling it as food. The product became known as Crisco®. Its name is derived from the initial sounds of "crystallized cottonseed oil." And so it began; 'trans fats' became a part of the American diet.

While there are beneficial trans-fats found in nature, such as conjugated linoleic acid (CLA), nature did not have a hand in making harmful manufactured trans fats. Harmful trans fats are man-made from artificially hydrogenated oils. They are produced when liquid vegetable oils are turned into solid fats through a process called hydrogenation. They have been a part of our diets now for over 100 years, but it has been just recently that we have begun to realize how deadly they are. There is no safe level.

Cities, towns, and even entire countries are banning trans fats. New York City was one of the first in the U.S. to ban the use of them in the cities' eateries. Montgomery County, Maryland was the first county to approve a ban on partially hydrogenated oils. California became the first state to ban trans fats in restaurants. They have been banned entirely in Denmark, Switzerland, and Austria. Yet, trans fats remain in over 60,000 food products.

Trans fats have been linked to depression, infertility, obesity, Alzheimer's disease, heart disease, liver dysfunction, cancer, reduced immune function, and diabetes.

Depression: Spanish researchers analyzed the diets of 12,059 people over a six year period and found those who ate the most trans fats had a 48% higher risk of depression than those who did not eat trans fats (Roan, 2011).

Infertility in Women: One 2007 study discovered that, "Each 2% increase in the intake of energy from trans fats, as opposed to that from carbohydrates, was associated with a 73% greater risk of ovulatory infertility..." (Chavarro, 2007). Trans fats pass from a pregnant woman's placenta to her unborn child. The unborn child's metabolism is adversely affected by trans fats in proportion to the amount consumed by the mother. Lactating mothers who consume substantial amounts of trans fats have less cream in their breast milk, since trans fats can lodge in the cellular spaces normally reserved for fatty acids. The cream is essential for maximum brain development of an infant. Increased dietary intake of trans fatty acids has also been associated with an increased risk of fetal loss.

Obesity: In June 2006, researchers at Wake Forest University reported after a six-year study, that calories from trans fats made laboratory monkeys fatter than calories from other forms of fat (Reed Business Information Ltd, 2006). In spite of efforts to prevent the monkeys from gaining weight by placing them on a low calorie diet, they gained it due to trans fat consumption.

Alzheimer's Disease: A study published in *Archives of Neurology* in February 2003, suggested that the intake of trans fat promotes the development of Alzheimer's disease (Morris, 2003).

C-reactive Protein (CRP): CRP is a known inflammation marker that, when elevated, predicts cardiovascular disease. A study of over 700 nurses showed that those in the highest quartile of trans fat consumption had blood levels of CRP that were 73% higher than those in the lowest quartile (Lopez-Garcia, 2005).

Liver Dysfunction: Trans fats are metabolized differently by the liver than other fats and interfere with delta-6 desaturase. Delta-6 desaturase is an enzyme needed to convert essential fatty acids to arachidonic acid and prostaglandins, both of which are important for cell function (Mahfouz, 1981).

Cancer: The European Prospective Investigation into Cancer and Nutrition suggests that the risk of breast cancer increases by 75%, due to increased intake of trans fat (Chajes, 2008).

Margarine is a popular trans fat. The manufacturing of this fake butter begins with cheap vegetable oils. These oils have already most likely been rendered harmful by the extraction process, which involves high temperatures and petrochemical solvents, such as benzene. One of the oils used comes from cottonseed. Cotton is not considered a food crop, so it can be highly sprayed with pesticides. In fact, it is the most highly sprayed crop in the world.

First, the oil is subjected to extremely high temperatures and pressure. Then, hydrogen is forced into a trans isomeric molecular structure to harden it. This process requires toxic substances, such as nickel oxide, which act as catalysts that enable the chemical change. The final product is a gray, smelly, greasy mass. Now it must be deodorized, again using high heat and chemical additives. This gray grease is then bleached white and then dyed yellow. Finally, artificial flavors are mixed in to make it taste like butter. Is it any wonder trans fats are linked to cancer?

Mankind has been consuming nature's fats, such as butter, lard, and coconut oil for thousands of years. Yet, heart disease only became common after 1920, when more people started to consume less expensive trans fats. Dr. Walter Willett, a professor of epidemiology and nutrition at Harvard Medical School, is a recognized authority on trans fats and has found that for every 4 to 5 grams of trans fat you eat, your risk of heart disease nearly doubles. To put that in perspective, some brands of microwave popcorn contain 14 grams of trans fat per bag. That is a big risk to take for a bag of popcorn.

The human enzyme lipase, which is responsible for breaking down fats in our bodies, is ineffective against lipids in the trans configuration. This means that trans fats remain in the blood stream for a much longer period of time, are prone to arterial deposition, and subsequent plaque formation.

The distortion of cell membranes, as well as cell structures, is perhaps one of the greatest dangers of trans fats. When the cells are affected, every part of the body is affected. In a healthy person, the cell membranes are made up of about 50% saturated fat. The saturated fats maintain the integrity of our cell membranes by keeping them stiff, yet flexible. This ensures that the cells function smoothly in assimilating nutrients, eliminating toxins, and keeping out pathogens. People who eat large amounts of trans fats have been found to have cell membranes that contain up to 20% trans fat. Once in your cell membrane, trans fats cannot be removed. Cells made up of trans fat, instead of saturated fat, become distorted and weak. Robert Erdmann, Ph.D., states that when the integrity of cell membranes is reduced, the lungs, digestive tract, and internal cells wind up "admitting allergens, undigested foods, viruses, and even potential carcinogens."

If the integrity of the cells is badly damaged to the point where the cell membranes do not interact chemically as they should, the body's immune system may no longer recognize them. This could lead to an immune reaction against the body's own tissues.

Research has shown that trans fats are incorporated into brain cell membranes and the myelin sheath, which could worsen the symptoms of fibromyalgia. They can also affect the brain in another way. Omega-3, an essential fatty acid, is vital for brain function. Trans fats are known to deplete the body's stores of omega-3, as well as its utilization.

Since trans fats accumulate, the poisoning is cumulative. Furthermore, there are no immediate visible effects of consuming trans fats. As a result, the warning signs are missed until the damage is done years later.

An article published in *The Journal of Nutritional Biochemistry* states that trans fats can also cause endothelial dysfunction (Chen, 2011). As we have discussed, the endothelial cells are already under attack in fibromyalgia.

Trans fats are not something to enjoy in moderation. As Tommy G. Thompson, Secretary of Health and Human Services for the U.S. Government stated during a trans fat press conference in 2003, "Trans fat is bad fat. The less trans fat people eat, the healthier they will be" (US Dept. of Health and Human Services, 2003). Trans fats have no business being in our food in the first place, so your goal should be to eliminate them entirely.

On July 10, 2002, the U.S. Government's advisor on health policy, the Institute of Medicine at the National Academy of Sciences, reported that manufactured trans fats are an ingredient that has *no safe level for human consumption* (Food and Nutrition Board, Institute of Medicine of the National Academies, 2005). Dr. Jeffrey Aron, M.D., University of California, San Francisco professor of medicine, and one of the nation's leading experts on fatty acids, calls trans fats, "One of the worst hidden dangers in the food supply." The American Medical Association supports any state and federal efforts to ban the use of artificial trans fats in U.S. restaurants and bakeries. The FDA still allows trans fats in our food due to the enormous influence of the food and oil industries. Consequently, you must be responsible for safeguarding your own health.

In order to avoid trans fats, you will need to read the ingredient list on all food labels. Even if the food label states, "Trans Fat: 0 grams," and even if the product advertises zero grams on the front label, it may still contain trans fats. How is that possible? The FDA only requires food companies to list trans fat content if the food contains 0.5 grams or more of it per serving. What this means is, if a food contains 0.49 grams of trans fat in one serving, that food will have "Trans Fat: 0 grams" listed in its nutrition facts.

This FDA loophole can be very misleading to the consumer. First, few people ever eat one serving of anything. So, if someone happened to eat two servings of a food that contained 0.49 grams of trans fat per serving, they would have eaten just under one full gram of trans fat. Of course, anything can have 'zero' grams using this method by simply reducing the size of the serving.

A quote from the FDA's website explaining how a consumer can tell if a product contains trans fats states, "Consumers can know if a food contains trans fats by looking at the ingredient list on the food label. If the ingredient list includes the words, "*Shortening, Partially Hydrogenated Vegetable Oil, or Hydrogenated Vegetable Oil*," the food contains trans fat" (U.S. Department of Health and Human Services, 2011).

The fats found in raw dairy and meat will help you heal, but trans fats, on the other hand, will bring your progress to a halt. Thomas Anderson, Ph.D., explains the difference, "It's important to understand that trans fats and saturated fats are completely different from one another and actually have opposite effects on health. The food industry's latest trick is to imply that both are 'bad' and should be avoided. This is a very dangerous deception, given that the fats in fresh meats and dairy food are important nutritionally. They lower the most significant risk factors for heart disease including blood pressure, lipoprotein, and homocysteine. These foods also raise protective HDL and they reduce the risk for inflammatory related disorders, such as asthma and arthritis. The only fats we truly need to be worried about are the oils made into margarine and shortening and used for deep frying. These are added fats, they are not part of any natural food, and they are the only fats ever linked to any disease."

Products that typically contain trans fats include:

- crackers
- cookies
- cake mixes
- pizza dough
- granolas
- frozen snacks (pizza, pot pies, burritos, etc.)
- margarine
- Crisco®
- candy bars
- fast food

- cupcake and cake icings
- microwave popcorns
- fried foods
- soups
- Cool Whip®
- ice cream
- potato chips
- packaged cheeses
- hot chocolate mixes
- doughnuts

A Processed-Food Future

The American College of Rheumatology estimates that between 6 million and 12 million people in the U.S. have fibromyalgia, and those numbers are rising. Autoimmune diseases, such as lupus and rheumatoid arthritis, are also rising.

Our western diets are no longer based on whole, living foods. They consist of processed foods laden with strange sounding chemicals and ingredients your body doesn't recognize and cannot utilize. At the very minimum, they will not cause you to get instantly ill, but they offer nothing your body can use to complete the startling array of metabolic processes required for you to stay alive and disease free.

Processed foods not only do not provide vital enzymes and bacteria, they strain and deplete the entire digestive tract. If you eat something that is completely devoid of vitality, your body will need to give up its stores of enzymes and energy to process it. In addition, the chemical residues in processed food will cause your liver and kidneys to work extra hard to protect your cells from the poisons they contain.

Many people will read this book and think that switching to a healthier diet is too expensive. We, as consumers, want cheap food, and the food industry has been doing a great job of complying with these demands. The reasons we are sick are not entirely the food industry's fault. However, we still pay for that choice, with higher insurance premiums, medical bills, medications, missed work days, and with our precious health and vitality.

Just as chronic disease is increasing, so is the earlier mortality of our children. Ours is the first generation where our children will not live as long as we do. If we fail to recognize the close connection between our food and our health, and don't start demanding better choices for us and our children, the future will only continue to grow dimmer.

Story of a 23-Year-Old: A Glimpse of the Future

Yesterday, a 23-year-old young man sat at my kitchen counter. He asked me if I knew how to get rid of arthritis. "Who has arthritis?" I asked.

"I do," he replied. He proceeded to tell me how stiff and painful his hands would often get. I told him it could be related to his diet. "What have you eaten today?" I asked. It was 5:00 p.m.

He said, "Well, I had some crackers for breakfast and I just had a cheeseburger and a pop."

"That could be your answer," I said. "Do you eat foods that contain enzymes?"

I knew from the blank look on his face that he didn't know what I was talking about. I told him enzymes were found in foods like fruits, vegetables, raw milk, and kefir.

"I drink a lot of milk," he said.

I went to my refrigerator and took out a green smoothie (I will tell you about these later) that I hadn't blended yet. I pointed out the beautiful colors and the ginger and the kiwi; both loaded with enzymes. I blended it for him to try.

"Not bad." he said.

"If you continue to eat the way you are, your arthritis will only get worse," I told him. "You are 23; this shouldn't happen to you at 23. Not at any age really."

I plan to give him a copy of this book. He might not be quite ready to change his diet, but I'm sure the day will come.

CHAPTER 20

Disease Management Is "Big Money Business"

GOING TO YOUR DOCTOR FOR A PRESCRIPTION if you are sick may seem like the right way to heal yourself. It's the way we've been taught, but many medications will only continue to damage your fragile digestive system, and will not allow you to heal. Healing you, however, may not be the number one priority of pharmaceutical companies.

You can read about this in Melody Peterson's book, *Our Daily Meds*. Here is an excerpt: "In this profit-driven world of medicine, I did not often hear the executives talk of cures. Instead, they focused like honeybees circling a picnic cake on products for what they called the chronic disorders. These were the drugs that did not cure, but 'managed' disease as patients took them once a day for the rest of their lives."

These 'management medications' cause direct destruction of enzymes, essential nutrients, and beneficial bacteria. They are also associated with severe side effects.

Big Money Business

(from Peterson, M. former medical reporter for *The New York Times*; author of *Our Daily Meds*)

Americans now spend over $200 billon a year on prescription drugs and this spending continues to increase by an average of 12 percent each year. Drugs are now the fastest growing part of the staggeringly-high American health care bill. Profits are soaring for drug companies, as the top 10 companies reported combined profits of $35.9 billion in 2002. This is more than all the rest of the 490 Fortune 500 companies put together! These same 10 companies spent $36 billion on advertising and marketing in 2002.

It seems the more they advertise, the more they rake in. But drugs have to be expensive, right? All that money for research and development has to come from somewhere. Don't believe it. In reality, in 2002 (the date of an extensive nonprofit investigation), only about 14 percent of Fortune 500 drug company revenues were applied toward research and development. Over 30 percent were devoted toward marketing and administration. Around 17 percent was received as profit. The Families USA, a nonprofit organization, reports the former CEO of Bristol- Meyers Squibb made $74,890,918 in 2001. This doesn't include his $76,095,611 of unexercised stock options. The chairman of Wyeth Pharmaceuticals made over $40 million, exclusive of an additional $40 million in stock options! Remember this when you wonder why your health insurance premiums continue to rise.

FIBROMYALGIA MEDICATIONS

Some common medications used to treat fibromyalgia are Cymbalta® (duloxetine), Savella® (milnacipran) Neurontin® (gabapentin), and Lyrica® (pregabalin).

Fibromyalgia Medications

- Duloxetine (Cymbalta®) is a selective *serotonin and noradrenaline* reuptake inhibitor antidepressant. Reuptake is the reabsorption of a neurotransmitter after it has performed its function of transmitting a neural impulse.

- Milnacipran (Savella®) is also a selective *serotonin and noradrenaline* reuptake inhibitor.

- Gabapentin (Neurontin®) is structurally related to the inhibitory neurotransmitter *gamma-aminobutyric acid (GABA).*

- Pregabalin (Lyrica®) was designed as a more potent successor to gabapentin. Pregabalin is a structural derivative of *GABA*. In cultured neurons prolonged application of pregabalin increases the density of *GABA* transporter protein and increases the rate of functional *GABA* transport.

As you can see, these medications are acting on some of the neurotransmitters (serotonin, noradrenaline, and GABA) that we have shown are involved in the disease process of fibromyalgia. These medications may delay or mask certain symptoms found in fibromyalgia, but they are associated with severe side effects that could worsen the disease process overall.

Low levels of serotonin, noradrenaline, and GABA are all a result of a lack of protease. The restoration of protease would address the actual cause of these missing neurotransmitters without the risk of side effects. These medications may also lead to further damage of the digestive tract, which could hinder or prevent recovery. For instance, some of the gastrointestinal side effects associated with Neurontin® are:

NEURONTIN®: Gastrointestinal Side Effects

(from www.fda.gov)

- Anorexia
- Flatulence
- Gingivitis, glossitis, gum hemorrhage
- Thirst
- Stomatitis
- Increased salivation
- Gastroenteritis
- Hemorrhoids, bloody stools
- Dysphagia
- Eructation
- Pancreatitis
- Peptic ulcer
- Colitis
- Blisters in mouth
- Tooth discolor
- Perlèche
- Salivary gland enlargement
- Lip hemorrhage
- Esophagitis
- Hiatal hernia
- Hematemesis
- Proctitis
- Irritable bowel syndrome
- Rectal hemorrhage
- Esophageal spasm
- Dyspepsia
- Dry mouth
- Constipation
- Dental abnormalities
- Increased appetite

Lyrica®: Side Effects
(from Lyrica.com, 2012)

- Serious, even life-threatening, allergic reactions
- Suicidal thoughts or actions
- Swelling of your hands, legs and feet
- Dizziness
- Sleepiness
- Blurry vision
- Weight gain
- Trouble concentrating
- Dry mouth
- Feeling high

Cymbalta®: Side Effects
(from www.cymbalta.com and www.drugs.com, 2012)

- Itching, right upper-belly pain, dark urine, yellow skin/eyes, or unexplained flu-like symptoms, which may be signs of life-threatening liver problems. Severe liver problems, some fatal, have been reported
- High fever, confusion, stiff muscles, muscle twitching, or racing heart rate, which may be signs of serotonin syndrome, a potentially life-threatening condition
- Abnormal bleeding, especially if Cymbalta® is taken with aspirin, NSAID pain relievers (like ibuprofen or naproxen), or blood thinners
- Serious, possibly life-threatening skin reactions, which may include skin blisters, peeling rash, mouth sores, hives, or other allergic reactions
- Abnormal mood (mania), which may include greatly increased energy, severe trouble sleeping, racing thoughts, talking more or faster than usual, and reckless behavior

(continued on next page)

CYMBALTA®: Side Effects
(continued)

- Seizures or convulsions
- Decreased blood pressure upon standing, which can cause dizziness or fainting, mostly when first starting or increasing the dose. Cymbalta can also increase blood pressure. Your healthcare provider should check your blood pressure prior to and while taking Cymbalta
- Headache, weakness or feeling unsteady, confusion, problems concentrating, or memory problems, which may be signs of low sodium levels in the blood. Elderly people may be at greater risk
- Problems with urination, including decreased flow or inability to pass any urine
- Changes in appetite or weight. Children and adolescents should have height and weight monitored

SAVELLA®: Side Effects
(from www.savella.com and www.drugs.com, 2012)

- Mood or behavior changes
- Anxiety, panic attacks
- Trouble sleeping
- Impulsive, irritable, agitated, hostile, aggressive, restless, hyperactive (mentally or physically), more depressed
- Thoughts about suicide or hurting yourself
- Pounding heartbeats or fluttering in your chest
- Painful or difficult urination
- Easy bruising or bleeding, nosebleeds, bloody or tarry stools, coughing up blood
- Severe weakness, seizure (convulsions)

(continued on next page)

Savella®: Side Effects
(continued)

- Chills or goose bumps, memory problems, trouble concentrating, agitation, hallucinations, fast heart rate, overactive reflexes, nausea, vomiting, diarrhea, loss of coordination fainting
- Very stiff (rigid) muscles, high fever, confusion, fast or uneven heartbeats, tremors, feeling like you might pass out, high blood pressure (severe headache, blurred vision, buzzing in your ears, chest pain, shortness of breath, uneven heartbeats)
- Stomach pain, loss of appetite, dark urine, clay-colored stools, jaundice (yellowing of the skin or eyes)

It would seem to make so much more sense to treat the problem at its source, rather than risk the serious side effects associated with various management medications.

CHAPTER 21

Choose Organic

THERE IS CONTINUOUS DEBATE over whether organic foods are really any better than non-organic foods. Are they worth the higher price tag that we pay? For the fibromyalgia sufferer, the answer is an unequivocal "yes." To make the point, I want to share with you the chemicals in one bag of non-organic popcorn.

List of Chemicals Found in
Non-Organic Popcorn Popped in Oil

(from the US FDA September 2003 Total Diet Study, page 12-13:
US Food and Drug Administration Total Diet Study – December 2006)

Summary of pesticide analytical results in food from the Food and Drug Administration's Total Diet Study program summarized by residue. Information pertains to (representative purchasable products) collected between September 1991 and October 2003.

- P-methaxychlor
- Chloroform
- Diclorobenzene
- Diazinon
- Methyl-pirimiphos

- 1,2,4-trimethylbezene
- Malthion
- Syrene
- Chlordane
- Trichicreethylene
- Benezene
- Cis-permethrin
- Xylene
- Trans-permethrin
- Polychlorinated biphenyls
- Ethylbenzene
- 1,11 trichloroethane
- Trans-chlorclane
- Toxaphene
- Cis-chlordane
- Chloropyrifos
- Dieldrin
- 1,1,1,2, tetrachloroethane
- Linclane

Not long ago, I had a man named Jim come to me for advice about a liver condition with which he suffers. I recommended some herbal teas and gave him some suggestions about his diet. I knew it would be an uphill battle on getting him to eat organic fruits and vegetables. When you suffer from a liver condition, eating organically is especially important because your liver is your detoxifying organ. He would nod his head in agreement when I would bring it up, but I knew I wasn't getting through to him.

One summer day, Jim stopped by while I was freezing some organic peaches for my winter smoothies. "Oh," he said, "I did the same thing this morning."

"Really," I said, knowing there were no organic peaches available in town at the moment.

"Where did you get them?"

"Safeway," he replied.

"Were they organic?" I asked.

"No," he smiled sheepishly.

"Do you know where they came from?" I asked.

"California, I think," he replied.

"Let me show you something." I went and retrieved my computer and set it on the kitchen counter. I brought up a government database on the amount of chemicals applied *per acre* for peaches in California (www.pesticideinfo.org). There were 50 listed. I then asked him to randomly pick a chemical from the list. We looked up the chemical on another government database. It said if you ingest the chemical, you should call a poison control center. At random, I have picked five of the pesticides, from the list of 50, to show what they are and what health risks they are associated with.

Common Pesticides Used on California Peaches and Their Health Risks

Pesticide	Uses	Health Risks
1,3-Dichloropropene	Fumigant, Nematicide	-PAN Bad Actor* -Acute Toxicity -Carcinogen -GroundWater Contaminant
Ziram	Fungicide, Microbiocide, Dog and Cat Repellent	-PAN Bad Actor* -Possible Carcinogen -Moderate Acute Toxicity -Developmental or or Reproductive Toxin -Suspected Endocrine Disruptor

(continued on next page)

Copper Sulfate (basic)	Fungicide, Algaecide, Molluscicide	-Moderate Acute Toxcity
Copper Hydroxide	Fungicide, Algaecide, Molluscicide	-Slight Acute Toxicity
Copper Oxide (ous)	Herbicide	-Moderate Acute Toxicity

* PAN Bad Actors are chemicals that are one or more of the following: highly acutely toxic, cholinesterase inhibitor, known/probable carcinogen, known groundwater pollutant, or known reproductive or developmental toxicant.

He leaned back in his chair, paused, and then said, "I've been poisoning myself my entire life."

I knew, for the rest of his life, he would choose organic if he possibly could, and so should you. For fibromyalgia sufferers, it is essential to choose organic produce that does not contain chemicals that will destroy enzymes. *Pesticides are poisons, and most poisons work by specific inhibition of enzymes.*

Researchers are finding a link between exposure to pesticides and an increased risk of developing rheumatoid arthritis (RA) and lupus. We have discussed the close association between fibromyalgia, RA, and lupus. The following press release is from the American College of Rheumatology.

RA and Lupus With Increased Exposure to Insecticides. Spraying for Bugs Could Increase Autoimmune Disease Risk: Press Release

(from Latimer, E. 2009. American College of Rheumatology)

PHILADELPHIA – Insecticide exposure may increase the risk of developing two well-known autoimmune rheumatic diseases in post-menopausal women, according to research presented this week at the American College of Rheumatology Annual Scientific Meeting in Philadelphia, Pa.

Farming and agricultural pesticide exposure has been linked to the development of rheumatoid arthritis and lupus, but it is unclear whether pesticide exposure in other settings might also increase risk of disease. The researchers believe these findings suggest that exposure to insecticides may increase the risk of developing RA or lupus in the general population, not only in the farming environment.

Personal Care Products and Indoor Air Pollution

Fibromyalgia patients also need to be especially careful about what they inhale and put on their skin. Many of the chemicals found in personal care products, dryer sheets, laundry detergents, air fresheners, and household cleaners are known carcinogens. These chemicals will also need to be detoxified by our bodies enzyme detoxification system (cytochrome P450), which will further deplete vitamin B12 and iron.

The Environmental Working Group (EWG), a public interest research group and advocacy organization, has found that more than one-third of all personal care products contain at least one known carcinogen. The average woman is exposed to 126 such chemicals on a daily basis. Sixty percent of everything we put on our skin is absorbed directly into our bloodstream, so we want to make sure to use products that are safe.

According to the Environmental Protection Agency (EPA), indoor pollution is one of the greatest health threats of our time. A five-year EPA study of over 600 households revealed that contaminant levels in the average home are up to 70 times higher than those found outdoors. Dryer sheets, synthetic fragrances, air fresheners, aerosol sprays, and perfumes are all contributing to this toxic indoor air pollution.

The EWG has an interactive product safety guide called Skin Deep at www.ewg.org that ranks over 15,000 name-brand products. The products you choose to use in your home and personal care should have a rank of zero. There is no need to use a product if it is hazardous to any degree. There are many safe alternatives available.

CHAPTER 22

Pure Proteins

IN ORDER TO RECOVER FROM FIBROMYALGIA, you will need to eat animal protein, and you will need to be able to digest it properly. You can't just go to Walmart®, however, and buy a steak for dinner. Your proteins will need to be free of antibiotics and hormones, and they must have been raised the way nature intended them to be. If the animal wasn't raised on pasture, then the eggs or meat will contain little to no vitamin B12. Vitamin B12 is made by organisms in the soil. An animal ingests vitamin B12 by grazing on pasture.

You will be paying a little more for pure proteins, but it will be money well spent. This is medicine for your body. If you needed a drug to keep your heart pumping, most likely you would not mind paying a little more for a drug that was free of contaminants. Not just any drug would do, and not just any protein will do.

LET'S START WITH FISH

Do you eat fish because you think it's healthy and is a rich source of vital omega-3s? How about salmon? Where does your salmon come from? Would you be surprised to learn that farmed salmon is perhaps the most contaminated food on supermarket shelves? According to British government advisors, it is the most toxic food you can consume. In every batch they tested, the salmon contained at least three toxic chemicals: DDT, dieldrin, and hexachlorobenzene. Pollutants concentrate in farmed salmon because they are fed fish pellets and oils that are themselves contaminated.

"Farmed salmon is the worst of the worst of all foodstuffs tested for DDT, dieldrin, and other cancer-causing chemicals. It is a contaminated product," stated Don Staniford, author of the article "Exposing the Salmon Industry" (Edwards, 2002).

And that pretty orange color? Where does it come from? It's a dye. Farmed salmon is gray. Wild salmon is orange because the salmon eat a natural diet of krill (tiny shrimp). The dye is in the pellets given to the salmon. It is called canthaxanthin and it has been linked to human eye defects and retinal damage. Don't be fooled by the term "Atlantic" salmon. That doesn't mean it came from the Atlantic Ocean, it is the breed of fish. In fact, that is the breed that is most often farmed.

For someone with fibromyalgia, there is another issue. Farmed salmon are fed huge amounts of antibiotics, which will destroy healthy intestinal flora. Antibiotics are needed to control the spread of infection in the high-density conditions of factory fish farming. In addition, the antibiotics we ingest in our foods from factory farming operations, as well as the antibiotics that go into our water supply, are believed to be a contributing factor to the growing antibiotic resistance problem in the U.S.

Fish can be healthy or extremely harmful. After learning how toxic some fish can be, I began sourcing it carefully from Alaska. I eat wild salmon, black cod, and halibut. Most of my fish comes from the deepest, coldest parts of the waters around Alaska. Sadly, our streams, lakes, and oceans are no longer the safe, clean sources of food they once were. We need to be extremely cautious when sourcing our fish.

CHICKEN

Do you think it would be a good idea to eat arsenic? Most anyone would answer, "No!" It would poison you, right? In fact, the scientific definition of arsenic is, "A highly poisonous element having three allotropic forms, yellow, black, and grey. Arsenic and its compounds are used in insecticides, weed killers, and various alloys. Atomic number 33" (American Heritage Science Dictionary, 2005).

Arsenic and its compounds are especially potent poisons. To deliberately add it to any food meant for human consumption would be irresponsible. And yet, arsenic is added to animal feed, particularly in the U.S., as a method of disease prevention and growth stimulation. For example, roxarsone is an arsenic-containing compound that has been used as a broiler starter by about 70% of the broiler growers since 1995 (Jones, 2007). Broiler chickens are a type of chicken specifically raised for meat production. The Poison-Free Poultry Act of 2009 proposed to ban the use of roxarsone in swine and poultry production.

Researchers from the National Institutes of Health and the USDA's Food Safety Inspection Service looked at 5,000 broiler chicken samples and found alarmingly high levels of arsenic contamination (Taylor, 2004). The amount of arsenic found in the broiler chickens greatly exceeded the Environmental Protection Agency's (EPA) upper safety limit of arsenic allowed in drinking water. The level of arsenic in the chicken sampled was six to nine times that allowed by the EPA.

The animals Americans eat are so heavily infested with internal parasites that adding arsenic to the feed can result in a "stunning increase in growth rates," says Donald Herman, a former Environmental Protection Agency researcher who has studied this use of arsenic for a decade. "They [the poultry industry] have tried everything to refrain it from becoming public knowledge," he stated.

The poultry industry argues that the organic form of arsenic given to chickens isn't toxic. The researchers, however, found not only elevated levels of organic arsenic in chicken meat; they found elevated levels of the highly toxic, inorganic form typically used only in insecticides and weed killers. Inorganic arsenic is a human carcinogen linked to liver, lung, skin, kidney, bladder, and prostate cancers. It can also cause metabolic, neurological, cardiovascular, gastrointestinal, and immune system abnormalities.

Arsenic is poison. Most poisons work by specific inhibition of enzymes. Commercial chicken is also heavily laden with antibiotics; another saboteur to your goal of restoring your gut flora. You can eat chicken; just make sure it is organic, pastured chicken.

EGGS

Not all eggs are created equal. Most people would naturally assume that if they purchased organic free range eggs, they would be making a healthy choice. I was one of those people. I used to buy organic free range eggs from my local supermarket. As I became more educated about the benefits of hens raised on pasture, and the dramatic increase in the egg's nutrition, I decided to do a little more research into the eggs I had been buying.

There was a phone number on the egg carton, so one day I called it. A nice sounding man answered the phone. I asked him if he could answer a few questions, since I had some health conditions and needed to be careful in my choice of eggs.

"Sure," he replied.

"To start with," I said, "How many chickens do you have?"

"Sixty thousand," he said.

I was shocked. "You have 60,000 chickens and they're all on pasture?"

"Oh, no, no," he answered. "The USDA definition of free range is they just have to have access to the out of doors. Our chickens are kept in big steel buildings with a concrete floor. We have two doors at the end of each building with a 5 by 5 ft. concrete paddock at either end. To be honest with you, they never go out there because we don't put food out there."

These chickens had never eaten a blade of grass in their lives. They had never taken a dust bath, which is their natural way to bathe. They had never taken a sun bath either, which would give their eggs natural vitamin D. They weren't in cages, but this was not a healthy environment for a chicken and these were not healthy eggs. If a chicken is never exposed to fresh air, sunlight, and soil, then their eggs will be lacking some very essential nutrients that we depend on for our health. The first of which would be vitamin B12.

Vitamin B12 comes from the soil, and animals need some of their food from the soil in order to ingest B12. In a natural environment, chickens scratch all day long in the soil for worms and bugs, and eat clover and other greens with soil particles attached. This is also important to keep in mind when you buy chicken to eat. Has it been truly pastured? If not, then the meat will not have B12 either. This, of course, is true of all land based animal proteins.

A study done by Mother Earth News found that eggs from hens raised on pasture may contain:

- 1/3 less cholesterol
- 1/4 less saturated fat
- 2/3 more vitamin A
- 2 times more omega-3 fatty acids
- 3 times more vitamin E
- 7 times more beta carotene

When I realized I would no longer be able to buy eggs from my local grocer, I began searching for an alternative local source. I wasn't very successful. I saw chickens that I was told were being pastured, which were actually being kept in dog runs with no grass whatsoever. I saw chickens with no feathers, huddled together in a totally dark building. I could find no one doing everything right. By that I mean, chickens being fed organic feed and allowed to roam freely on plenty of green grass. So, I got my own chickens. They are the most spoiled, pampered chickens on the planet, and they reward me with the most nutritious, delicious eggs I have ever tasted. At first, I was the only one in my neighborhood to have chickens, but after some of my neighbors met my chickens and tasted their eggs, they realized what they had been missing and got chickens of their own.

If eggs are going to be a part of your recovery, I would encourage you to be absolutely sure they come from truly pastured organic chickens. The only way to do this is to visit your source. Do the chickens look healthy? Are they being fed organic grains? What about cleanliness? Or, maybe you could just get your own chickens, as I did.

Your local farmers' market is a good place to look for fresh organic eggs. Online resources, such as www.localharvest.org and www.eatwild.com, can also help connect you with local organic farmers and ranchers.

WHERE'S THE BEEF?

The ideal beef for you to choose would be organic, pasture raised, and pasture finished. All cows start out on pasture, but most cows end up in feedlots. Cows were designed to eat grasses, not grains. They have a four-chambered stomach to ferment the grasses as they move through their digestive system. When you consume beef from cows that have eaten grass, you raise your conjugated linoleic acids (CLAs) or omega-3s. CLAs are potent inflammation fighters. When you eat beef that was fed an unnatural diet of grains, you will raise your omega-6 fatty acids, which in fact, promote inflammation.

The result of animals fed unnatural diets is that they get sick, and they do so almost immediately. To keep them alive until they are fat enough to slaughter, they are fed massive amounts of antibiotics. The Centers for Disease Control and Prevention (CDC) estimates that 50 million pounds of antibiotics are produced each year in the U.S., and about 40% of those antibiotics are used in livestock. Nearly 80% of farm animals receive sub-therapeutic levels of antibiotics in their feed, at least part of the time.

In addition to the huge amounts of antibiotics, they are fed a "hormone" cocktail. Today, ranchers routinely use six types of sex hormones. Testosterone, progesterone, and oestradiol-17 beta, are the "natural" sex hormones. Trembolone acetate, zeranol, and melengestrol acetate are the synthetic sex hormones. Like the steroids used by bodybuilders, these substances increase muscle and fat growth, making each cow heavier by about 50 pounds. They also make the animals grow faster, which allows them to be taken to market more quickly. Most of us would never take hormones without thoughtful consideration of the ramifications to our health. So why do many of us thoughtlessly eat these same hormones in the meat we consume?

This is not the whole story of beef, but for the purposes of your recovery, we will stop here and address what is relevant. Lack of antibiotics and hormones, high levels of omega-3s, and vitamin B12 are your very specific reasons to choose organic, pasture raised and finished beef.

Processed Meats

Consuming processed meats (hot dogs, sausage, bacon, lunch meats, etc.) can increase the risk of pancreatic cancer by a whopping 6,700%, according to a study conducted at the University of Hawaii (Nöthlings, 2005). This study followed 200,000 men and women for seven years. Additionally, leukemia rates skyrocket by 700% when a diet includes hot dogs. The World Cancer Research Fund (WCRF) has recently concluded that no amount of processed meat is safe. A previous analysis by the WCRF found that eating just one sausage a day raises your risk of developing bowel cancer by 20%.

Other studies have found that processed meats increase your risk of:

- colon cancer by 50 %
- bladder cancer by 59 %
- stomach cancer by 38 %

The culprit in these meats is the sodium nitrite (a preservative and coloring agent). Sodium nitrite is a precursor to highly carcinogenic nitrosamines. Nitrosamines are potent cancer-causing chemicals that accelerate the formation and growth of cancer cells throughout the body. We need to restore the function of the pancreas, not directly cause it harm. Cancer aside, there is no hot dog or bologna sandwich that is worth having fibromyalgia.

CHAPTER 23

Beverages

It is estimated that Americans get over 20% of their daily caloric intake from beverages. This significant percentage shows that what we drink is an important part of our overall diet and will have an impact on our recovery. We may not always make the best choices in our beverages, reaching for sodas, energy drinks, sugary coffees, etc. The beverages many of us drink need a makeover. The first and foremost is our water.

What's in the Water?

Fluoride: aka Hydrofluoric Acid

Fluoride is the ingredient that is in your toothpaste and that the dentist uses when you get your teeth cleaned. Fluoride is also the chemical they are dumping in our water supply, which we are drinking by the gallons. Fluoride is not an element found on the periodic table, but rather an industrial by-product of steel, cement, aluminum, phosphate, and nuclear weapons manufacturing. Instead of it being a horribly costly pollutant that needs to be disposed of properly, it has cleverly been turned into a multi-billion dollar a year industry. It is used to produce fluorocarbons and chlorofluorocarbons for freezers and air conditioners. Fluoride is also used in the manufacturing of computer screens, light bulbs, semiconductors, plastics, herbicides, and toothpaste. The Merck Index indicates that sodium fluoride is used primarily as a rat and cockroach poison and is also the active ingredient in most toothpaste.

Fluoride was believed, for a short time, to strengthen teeth. As a result, our government began adding it to our water supply to create strong healthy teeth in our children. However, for the last 50 years, study after study has shown that fluoride does not strengthen teeth, it actually does the opposite. Fluoride is so bioactive that it interferes with the reactions necessary for collagen production. The mineralization of collagen is what leads to bone production and strong teeth. By disrupting this reaction, fluoride has been linked to osteoporosis, fractures, calcium stones, and crystals in joints and organs. Fluoride also disrupts DNA, which can lead to premature aging and increased rates of cancer.

For someone suffering from fibromyalgia, fluoride is extremely harmful. Fluoride directly attacks the body's enzymes by changing their shape. Enzymes act like a lock and a key, fitting together to carry out the thousands of cell reactions that our bodies need for health and survival. Once an enzyme's shape is changed, it becomes ineffective and often dangerous.

The following abstract shows the association between the first outbreak of chronic fatigue syndrome and fluoride in the drinking water. The researchers state, "Fluoride is a potent enzyme poison due to its affinity towards trace minerals."

Chronic Fatigue, Fluoride, and Heavy Metals
(from Phelps, J.E. 2005)

The term "CFS" or Chronic Fatigue Syndrome made its national appearance in the mid 1980's with the investigations of Dr. Paul Cheney concerning sick persons in the area of Lake Tahoe. South Lake Tahoe has public water supplies from wells that have metal contamination, often associated with volcanic zones or mining. South Lake Tahoe water reports have specific caution for immune compromised persons because of these pollutants.

Cheney's patients were from an extinct volcanic zone with contaminates in well water. From the study of volcanology, we know volcanic zones have many of the toxic *fluorides* and metal problems associated with mining.

Fluoride is a potent enzyme poison due to its affinity toward trace minerals.

The Center for Disease Control (CDC) has advised anyone with a compromised immune system to consult his or her physician before drinking tap water. In addition, the *Clinical Toxicology of Commercial Products* handbook states, "Fluoride is more poisonous than lead and just slightly less poisonous than arsenic" (Gleason, 1957).

In his book, *Fluoride the Aging Factor*, Dr. Yiamouyiannis included a quote from a Proctor & Gamble® executive, saying, "A seven-ounce tube of toothpaste, theoretically at least, contains enough fluoride to kill a small child" (Yiamouyiannis, 1986). If you check your toothpaste packaging, the FDA now requires a warning be printed on the label. The warning states, "If more than used for brushing is accidentally swallowed, get medical help or contact a Poison Control Center right away." *Call Poison Control if you swallow your toothpaste?* Interestingly enough, the portion you use to brush your teeth (approximately 0.25 mg), contains the same amount of fluoride found in an average glass of tap water.

In addition to our water and toothpaste, there are numerous other sources of fluoride that we ingest. Some pesticides contain fluoride. After all, what kills rats and roaches would surely take out the pests that threaten our fruits and vegetables. Buying organic food is once again the obvious choice over fruits and vegetables that have been sprayed with pesticides.

How do we ingest fluoride?

- drinking water
- vegetables and fruit – fluoride contained in the pesticides and possibly the water with which they are watered
- toothpaste
- canned foods

- processed foods
- soft drinks
- beer

Additionally, a 1998 lab test done at Sequoia Analytical Labs showed very high concentrations of fluoride in the following (Jones, 1998):

- Dole Pineapple® canned
- Snapple®
- Coke Classic®
- Hansen's Soda®
- Minute Maid Orange Juice®
- Gerber Strawberry Juice® for babies
- Amstel Lite® beer
- Rice Dream® (rice milk)
- Sunny Delight® orange drink
- Pepsi®

Fluoride aside, you should not be consuming most of the things on the above list anyway. It is important to drastically decrease your intake of fluoride, as it can be a direct obstacle to restoring functioning enzymes to your system. Using home filtration systems, eliminating fluoridated beverages, and not using fluoridated toothpaste is a good place to start.

Ditch the fluoride and get a brighter, healthier, fresher mouth in return by making your own toothpowder.

TOOTHPOWDER

Ingredients:

- ¼ teaspoon organic powdered clove
- ¼ cup baking soda
- ½ teaspoon organic dried spearmint leaf
- ½ teaspoon sea salt

- ½ teaspoon organic dried sage
- ½ teaspoon organic dried peppermint leaf

Preparation:

Mix the above ingredients together in a blender or small food processor.

You know how after you shampoo your new carpet for the first time it seems to get dirtier faster? That's because a sticky, tacky residue was left on the carpet from the soap, which attracts dirt. The same thing is true of your toothpaste. If you use sticky, tacky toothpaste, your teeth will just attract dirt and bacteria. Our toothpowder leaves your teeth feeling clean, with no leftover residue. In addition, the herbs contain powerful antibacterial and breath-freshening properties that only nature can provide. Plus, you won't need to keep an emergency number handy, just in case you swallow some!

Chlorine

Chlorine is another toxic chemical that is added to our water supply. Chlorine has been linked to cancer, heart disease, and the potential for miscarriage and birth defects. Prolonged exposure has also been shown to increase the risk of rectal and bladder cancers.

The U.S. EPA defines chlorine as "a pesticide designed to kill living organisms." Should we be drinking this? Chlorine is used to kill harmful bacteria in our drinking water that may make us ill, but killing our own good bacteria, cells, and tissues is definitely making us sick too.

Even more surprising is where we get most of our chlorine exposure. We should not be drinking it or swimming in it, but should we be showering in it? It is estimated that 2/3 of our exposure comes from showering and bathing. The warm water opens our pores and our skin acts like a sponge soaking it in. Additionally, we inhale it as a steam. It is important to use a filter on your shower head, as well as for your drinking water.

The chlorine gas we inhale goes directly into our bloodstream and must be filtered out through the digestive system and the kidneys, which often are already overburdened. It has also been linked to increased bronchitis and asthma in children, which has increased 300% in the last two decades. Chlorine is a known carcinogen, but it also readily combines with other chemicals, forming some of the most environmentally hazardous chemicals known.

A form of chlorine, called dioxin, is produced as a by-product of the dye process for many of the things in our lives that are white. This includes writing paper, toilet paper, paper towels, Styrofoam® cups, and the inside of our milk cartons. A study reported in *Science News* found that the dioxin used to dye the inside of milk cartons leached into the milk (Raloff, 1988). Additionally, when you drink hot liquids from dioxin bleached cups, it leaches into the beverage.

Dioxins are endocrine disrupters. Your endocrine system consists of your ovaries, testes, parathyroid, thymus, thyroid, adrenals, organ tissue, and pancreas. Dioxins can interrupt the chemical signal process and severely compromise one's health.

COFFEE

I like coffee, *a lot*, and I don't feel guilty drinking it. It is a primary source of antioxidants in the American diet. Study after study proves it is healthy in moderate amounts.

There is one thing I insist on though, it must be organic. Most of the coffee grown in the world is sprayed with pesticides and fungicides containing dangerous chemicals. These chemicals, such as chlordane, chlorpyrifos, DDT, disulfoton, endsulfan, and methylparathion are so toxic to humans and wildlife that some of them have been banned from use in the United States. Among the adverse health effects of such chemicals are death, nerve poisoning, cancer, liver cirrhosis, sexual dysfunction, and more. When hot water is poured over the coffee beans, these chemicals are released into your morning cup. That's not coffee; that's a witch's brew, and that is no way to start your day.

CHAPTER 24

Yeast and Gluten

THERE IS A HIGH CORRELATION of gluten intolerance associated with fibromyalgia. Gluten is a protein and fibromyalgia sufferers are unable to properly break down proteins. This gluey protein is found in grains like barley, rye, and wheat. It can strip the villi (little fingers in the intestinal tract) causing malabsorption, which can lead to all sorts of problems. There is also a connection to lack of vitamin B12 and gluten intolerance. An important function of B12 is repairing damaged, flattened microvilli. With sufficient B12 in the bloodstream, the intestinal cells and microvilli can rejuvenate.

Research shows that patients with celiac disease are deficient in vitamin B12, which is evidence they are not breaking down animal proteins, in addition to gluten. The study entitled "Low serum vitamin B12 is common in celiac disease and is not due to autoimmune gastritis" concluded that, "Low B12 is common in celiac disease without concurrent pernicious anemia, and may be a presenting manifestation" (Dickey, 2002).

How did the 'staff of life' become something we should be concerned about eating? Remember what Jesus said, "Man must not live by bread alone." As described in the Bible, visualize his disciples walking through wheat fields and plucking off the tops of the wheat stalks to eat. So, what has changed? Not just the wheat itself, but the way bread is made.

Our ancestors, and virtually all pre-industrialized peoples, soaked or fermented their grains before making them into porridge or breads, etc. Fermenting grains through the use of sourdough yeast breaks down the proteins in the grain into a simpler form that is much more easily digested. A diet high in unfermented whole grains, particularly high-gluten grains like modern day wheat, puts an enormous strain on the digestive system.

Why did we stop making bread the traditional way? Convenience and money are both factors. Sourdough yeast lives forever if you take care of it. Once you have it, and you can easily get some from a friend that bakes sourdough bread, you never have to buy it again. So, where's the money in that? Fleischmann's first engineered "yeast that would die" around the 1860s as a convenience. Sourdough yeast takes longer to rise. The changeover became complete in the 1980s, when instant yeast was introduced. Once again, we've traded health and flavor for convenience.

What about someone who is gluten intolerant or has celiac disease? Would they actually be able to consume fermented bread with no toxic effects? The study entitled "Sourdough bread made from wheat and nontoxic flours and started with selected lactobacilli is tolerated in celiac sprue patients" showed that even someone with celiac disease can eat bread with no toxic effects, as long as the bread is properly fermented (Di Cagno, 2004). In the study, sourdough bread was made from 30% wheat and a mixture of oat, millet, and buckwheat flours. The bread was fed to 17 patients with celiac disease with no negative consequences. However, when the same 17 patients were fed the bread make with baker's yeast, 13 patients showed "a marked alteration in intestinal permeability."

In an additional study entitled "Safety for patients with celiac disease of baked goods made of wheat flour hydrolyzed during food processing" celiac patients were fed a 60-day diet of baked goods made from wheat flour manufactured with sourdough lactobacilli and fungal protease (Greco, 2011). They also experienced no ill effects.

For someone with fibromyalgia, eating bread (or grain) that has not been properly soaked or fermented will place an added burden on your already weak digestion. However, if you can find (or bake yourself) an organic, whole grain sourdough bread in your community, by all means, enjoy!

SOURDOUGH PANCAKES

These pancakes are easy and delicious; don't let the use of sourdough intimidate you.

Ingredients and Preparation:

The night before, mix well (to incorporate some air) 1 cup of your sourdough starter with 1 ½ cups of organic whole wheat flour and 1 cup of warm water (85°-90°). Cover bowl with plastic wrap and leave at warm room temperature (70°-85°) overnight.

The next morning, return 1 cup of the starter mixture to the fridge.

Then mix the remaining 1 ½ cups of starter with the following organic ingredients:

- 1 egg, slightly beaten
- 1 tablespoon of honey (or more if you like)
- 3 teaspoons of sea salt
- ½ teaspoon (generous) of baking soda
- 2 tablespoons of milk

Try to have your ingredients at room temperature. This will help to make the pancakes more tender. Bake on a 400° griddle. Enjoy!

Soaked Oatmeal

Oatmeal is one of our favorite breakfast foods. Loaded with fiber and antioxidants, oatmeal offers many health benefits, from stabilizing blood sugar to reducing the risk of cancer and heart disease. Research has also shown that oats can protect the gut from toxins that would otherwise lead to intestinal permeability, which would be especially beneficial for a fibromyalgia sufferer (Keshavarzian, 2001).

Overnight soaked oatmeal couldn't be easier or more delicious. You just soak raw organic quick oats overnight in raw milk or kefir. Then in the morning, add a little more milk and fruit (our favorite is strawberries), drizzle with honey, and you're ready to eat.

OVERNIGHT SOAKED OATMEAL

Ingredients and Preparation:

- 1 cup of organic quick oats
- Add ½ cup of raw milk and squish down oats
- Cover and put in the fridge overnight
- In the morning, add milk to suit, organic fruit, and some raw honey

CHAPTER 25

A Healthy Gut

A HEALTHY GUT IS HOME to thousands of species of beneficial bacteria that live along our digestive tract, from our mouths, to our stomachs, and throughout our intestines. They help us digest our food, synthesize vitamins, and are vital for the proper functioning of our immune system. They work together synergistically and each species plays a vital and necessary role. You have likely heard of lactobacillus and acidophilus, but what about the other 750 trillion bacteria, yeast, and other microorganisms that are believed to inhabit a healthy person's body? These diverse micro-floras comprise three to five pounds of a person's body weight. They are all living, vital organisms that only nature can create and sustain. Man has not been able to even identify all of the species, let alone create them. These living bacteria don't come in a bottle or a pill. They come from food that is living, whole, complex, and in perfect balance.

One of the reasons you are sick is because you have lost the beneficial bacteria that you were designed to have. If all the bacteria in the world died it would not be long before all life on earth ceased to exist.

When we are sick, we often look to antibiotics, which kill bacteria, to become healthy again. "Anti-biotic" means "against life," all life. They kill off all the bacteria in our gut, because they can't recognize the difference between the good bacteria and the bad. Only about five percent of our gut bacteria is pathogenic; the other 95% is beneficial and necessary for our survival. How do you fix that kind of destruction? By eating yogurt? Remember, there are thousands of species of beneficial bacteria. How many strains does pasteurized yogurt contain? The pasteurization process killed off all the original bacteria. The few strains present when you purchase the yogurt were added back in. They will not restore your gut to its original condition. Thankfully, nature has provided us with foods that will.

Just as factory farming is now the norm, the way we eat seems normal. That is not the way it used to be. Chickens on the family farm were free to search for bugs, grass, clover, or worms, and eat whatever else they found interesting. They took their baths in the sun and the dirt. They absorbed the sunlight and their bones stayed strong. The eggs had bright yellow-orange yolks filled with omega-3 fatty acids and contained 40 times more beta-carotene than a modern egg. The chickens were happy and healthy.

Our ancestors also ate fermented foods with their meals. And I don't mean our ancestors like cavemen ancestors. I mean just 100 years ago. The cellars of most homes were filled with raw fermented sauerkraut and pickles to last the winter. They drank fermented apple cider made in the fall and raw milk, kefir, and yogurt that they made daily. They snacked on raw cheese filled with enzymes and good bacteria. Their root cellars were filled with enzyme-rich fruits and vegetables like raw carrots, apples, and cabbage. In the summer, they ate vegetables and fruits from their gardens. These foods provided beneficial enzymes in abundance. They ate proteins too, including eggs and pastured meats, like beef, pork, and chicken. Our ancestors had the enzymes from the fermented foods they were eating to break down these proteins. Today, our diets do not include any of these enzyme-rich foods. Therefore, we are unable to properly break down the proteins we consume.

CHAPTER 26

Foods that Restore Beneficial Enzymes and Bacteria

WE WILL NEED TO RESTORE these beneficial foods to our diets, so that we too can properly metabolize proteins and give our bodies the nutrients they need to be healthy and disease free.

UNPROCESSED MILK (RAW MILK)

One vital source of enzymes is milk that has not been pasteurized, ultra-pasteurized, or homogenized. Is there a difference between the milk we drink today and the milk of the past? Dairy products have been consumed for thousands of years and are mentioned in the Bible as beneficial foods. Before pasteurization, milk was consumed in its raw form, and still is by many cultures. Even prior to refrigeration, raw milk did not spoil. It soured naturally and was made into butter or cultured into products like cheese, cottage cheese, kefir, and yogurt.

Modern milk, however, is the number one allergic food in the country. It is linked to so many of the ailments that raw milk can help alleviate. These ailments include:

- diarrhea/cramps/bloating
- gastrointestinal bleeding
- colic
- iron deficiency/anemia
- skin rashes and allergies
- osteoporosis
- tooth decay
- ear infections
- heart disease and atherosclerosis
- cancer
- type I diabetes
- arthritis
- rheumatoid arthritis
- autism
- excessive mucus production
- allergies
- rashes
- depression
- mood swings

What has happened to turn one of the most nutritious, virtuous beverages given to mankind into one of the most harmful? Your recovery will depend on you getting this one right. Raw milk is a vital, living food and medicine for our bodies. Raw milk, from cows that have been raised on pasture, is full of enzymes, amino acids, immunoglobulins (antibodies), metal-binding proteins (remember our discussion on zinc-binding proteins), vitamin binding proteins, several growth factors, and beneficial bacteria.

Raw milk contains over 60 known enzymes that have far-reaching effects in the body. Several enzymes in raw milk, including amylase, phosphatases, and lipases, break down starches, lactose, fats, and phosphate compounds, to make milk more digestible. Other enzymes, like catalase, lysozyme, and lactoperoxidase, help kill unwanted bacteria both in the milk and in our bodies. In fact, many people who are lactose intolerant, or even allergic to milk, experience no symptoms when they drink raw milk. This is because the enzymes are present to aid in digestion and assimilation of the key nutrients and minerals. One of these enzymes is lactase. Lactase is responsible for the digestion of lactose in milk. When milk is pasteurized, this enzyme is destroyed and people may experience "lactose intolerance" as a result.

During pasteurization, the milk is forcefully heated to high temperatures in a process that resembles nothing it would be exposed to in nature. This heating kills all the enzymes. In fact, the death of the enzymes is how they determine the process was successful. When all the enzymes are dead, the pasteurization process is complete. One of the missing enzymes, phosphatase, is necessary for the assimilation of calcium. So, drinking pasteurized milk does little to nothing in terms of building strong teeth and bones. There are 59 other missing enzymes that were meant for equally important functions within the human body.

Pasteurization also results in the loss and/or adulteration of vitamins A, D, and E. Up to 60% of these fat-soluble vitamins are lost. Vitamin C loss is upwards of 50%. *Vitamin B6 and B12 are completely destroyed.*

Lactoferrin is just one of the many proteins found in raw milk. Lactoferrin binds iron, contributing to increased absorption and assimilation. This protein is also said to have antibacterial activity against several species of bacteria that contribute to tooth decay. Conversely, pasteurized milk contributes to tooth decay and anemia, partially due to the lactoferrin being denatured and no longer able to perform its function.

The denaturing of proteins during the pasteurization process is of grave importance to the fibromyalgia sufferer. During pasteurization, proteins are deformed, denatured, and broken up in such a way that the body thinks they are foreign. The body will then mount an immune response against them.

Raw milk also contains 22 amino acids, including eight that are considered essential. This means our body relies on foods to obtain them because it cannot produce them on its own. Additionally, our bodies cannot store amino acids, meaning that it needs a continuous supply. If even one amino acid is missing or damaged, the rest cannot function properly.

Kurt Oster, Chief of Cardiology and Chairman of the Department of Medicine at Park City Hospital in Bridgeport, CT states, "Milk has been changed over the years by processing into an unrecognizable, physiochemical emulsion, which bears very little resemblance to original, natural, and nutritional milk."

Why is milk pasteurized if it doesn't benefit those who drink it? Pasteurization turns a living food into a dead one and enables the milk to sit on store shelves for months. We have seen milk in stores dated six months from the expiration. In the case of ultra-pasteurization, refrigeration isn't needed until it is opened. Basically, putting it in the refrigerated section is for show. Consumers would likely have an issue looking for their milk and creamer next to the potato chips. This extended shelf-life benefits the producers and suppliers of the milk, not the health of the consumer. If you switch to fresh raw milk from cows raised outside on green grass, you will benefit yourself, the cow, and the farmer who sold it to you.

Mark McAffee of Organic Pastures, a raw milk dairy, has sold thousands of gallons of milk with no ill effects reported. Independent tests were performed between McAffee's raw milk and commercial pasteurized milk. Disease pathogens, including salmonella, listeria, and E.coli, were added to both the raw and the pasteurized milk. The raw milk, which contains beneficial bacteria, would not support the growth of pathogens and they all died off. However, in the pasteurized milk, the pathogenic bacteria thrived and proliferated. In the absence of the beneficial bacteria, harmful bacteria can more easily take hold.

Adding raw milk to your food regime will be essential for healing your digestive tract and eventually your disease. Raw organic pastured goat's milk is equally as beneficial as cow's milk. For additional information on raw milk, you can visit www.realmilk.com. This is also a great site to find raw milk producers in your area.

Raw Cheese

One of the best foods you can eat to bring more enzymes, vitamin B12, and good bacteria into your diet is cheese made from organic unpasteurized milk. In order for the cheese to contain vitamin B12, the cows that produced the milk must have been raised on pasture. This is because vitamin B12 is found in soil.

It is also important to pay attention to what your cheese is wrapped in. You may make the effort to buy organic raw cheese, but then find it is wrapped in plastic. Consumer's Union scientists found that out of 19 cheddar cheese samples, the seven packed in clear polyvinyl chloride (PVC) plastic cling wrap, such as Reynold's®, Saran Wrap®, or Glad Cling Wrap®, contained the plasticizer DEHA at an average of 153 parts per million (ppm) (Groth, 1998). This far exceeds the 18 ppm limit on food migration set by the Commission of the European Communities for DEHA. DEHA has been linked to birth defects and liver cancer in lab animals. Most of the DEHA from the plastic wrap ended up in the cheese. In fact, plasticizer molecules can migrate from packaging into food until they are depleted. Migration begins immediately.

Frustrating, isn't it? We order our cheese from James Ranch. The ranch is set in one of the most beautiful, pristine environments you can imagine. The cheese comes in wheels that are sealed in wax. We slice the cheese as needed and place in glass lidded containers in the fridge for easy snacking. If you team up with friends or family who are taking this wonderful journey with you, you can share a wheel of cheese and shipping expenses.

Kefir

Kefir, which means "feel good" in Turkish, is an ancient, cultured, enzyme-rich food that is filled with friendly bacteria. It is made from whole organic raw milk and it will help you in ways nothing else can. Raw milk kefir is an essential part of your recovery. Here are some of the reasons why.

Although homemade yogurt is a perfectly healthy food, it doesn't hold a candle to kefir. Both are cultured milk products, but they work differently. The digestive enzymes in yogurt help digest the yogurt and only the yogurt. Kefir comes with extra enzymes that attach themselves to the walls of your gastrointestinal tract. The yogurt's nutrient delivery is gone in 24 hours, while kefir's is indefinite. It will fill your digestive tract with living, beneficial bacteria and enzymes.

Kefir contains 30-35 major strains of friendly bacteria not commonly found in yogurt. It is a turbo-charged, antibiotic colon cleanser. Kefir also contains beneficial yeasts, such as Saccharomyces kefir, which dominate and eliminate pathogenic yeasts. The beneficial yeasts penetrate the mucosal lining, where unhealthy yeast and bacteria reside, and destroy them. The friendly Candida yeast in kefir will kill the Candida albicans yeast that causes the classic yeast infection.

The complete proteins in kefir are partially digested and therefore more easily utilized by the body. Kefir is also rich in vitamin B12. You will have an immediate source of B12 to begin to heal. We cannot stress enough how important this is. Also, since the proteins are already partially digested, this will lessen the load on what little enzymes you are starting with. There just isn't another food out there that can match kefir for your specific needs.

Kefir also contains an ample supply of phosphorous, which aids your body in utilizing the proteins you are now able to break down for cell growth and energy. It is an excellent source of biotin, a B vitamin, which aids the body's absorption of other B vitamins (including B12). Kefir has a particularly calming effect on the nervous system. It contains calcium and magnesium, both of which are beneficial for healthy nerves and restful sleep. It also contains tryptophan, a precursor to serotonin and melatonin, well-known for their relaxing properties. What if you are lactose intolerant? The lactose in kefir has already been predigested by the beneficial bacteria in the kefir. Therefore, even people with milk sensitivities can usually drink it. This is nature's perfect food.

A man-made probiotic supplement in pill form has around 15 million bacteria. Yes, that sounds like a lot, but if you look at 500 ml. of kefir, you get up to five trillion beneficial bacteria! The most difficult part of making kefir will be locating a source for organic raw pastured milk. Store bought kefir is made from pasteurized milk and contains denatured proteins.

In addition to the raw cow's or goat's milk, you will need kefir grains (look in the resources section for where to order). Kefir grains are colonies of microorganisms, mostly yeasts and bacteria, that are beneficial to the human digestive tract. They form small, irregular, whitish balls, that when immersed in a nourishing liquid (usually raw milk), digest the liquid through a fermentation process that results in "kefir".

Once you have kefir grains, you then add the grains to the milk. Leave the milk on your kitchen counter overnight and you will have kefir within 1-2 days. Kefir resembles unsweetened yogurt in consistency and taste. Most likely you have never heard of kefir before reading this. It's just another casualty of our processed-food dependent generation. It has been consumed for centuries by some of the healthiest cultures in the world. You will soon be quite an expert in kefir and you will notice immediate improvements in your health and energy.

KEFIR

Preparation and Ingredients:

- Put your kefir grains* in a quart sized jar and add raw milk, leaving some room at the top for the kefir to expand.
- Gently stir the grains and the milk, cover with a paper towel, cheesecloth, or coffee filter, and rubber band.
- Allow to sit on the counter 24-48 hours stirring occasionally. It will take 1-2 days for the milk to thicken.
- When the curds have separated from the liquid whey (yellowish liquid), your milk kefir is ready. It should have approximately the same consistency as yogurt.
- Separate the kefir grains from the kefir to drink. Put kefir grains in a new jar and add milk to start the process anew.

* Kefir "grains" are not actually grains at all but colonies of beneficial bacteria and yeasts, along with some proteins and sugars. When placed in milk, the grains culture the milk making it into kefir. You will need to order your first set of raw milk kefir grains (see Resources section in the back) or get them from a friend. Once you have your grains, if cared for properly, they will last indefinitely.

That's it, you're done! I think it is best served very cold. I even chill my glass. Add fruit and honey, just as if you are making a smoothie. Enjoy!

If you have more questions about how to make kefir, you can visit our website: Nature Had It First http://www.naturehaditfirst.com/recipes/raw-milk-kefir-instructions/

Now that you have your homemade kefir you can use it for a variety of things, including a base for smoothies. Here are some of our favorite recipes:

STRAWBERRY-BANANA SMOOTHIE

Ingredients:

- Homemade kefir
- 1 cup of organic strawberries
- 1 organic banana
- Honey to taste (we use organic raw honey)
- 1 teaspoon organic vanilla extract
- Ice

Preparation:

Blend all the ingredients except for the kefir together. Add the kefir last and just give a quick stir to minimize the blending and denaturing of the proteins.

ORANGE-BANANA SMOOTHIE

Ingredients

- Homemade kefir
- 1 organic banana
- 1 organic orange or large tangerine
- Honey to taste (we use organic raw honey)
- 1 teaspoon organic vanilla extract (optional)
- Ice

Preparation:

Blend all the ingredients except for the kefir together. Add the kefir last and just give a quick stir to minimize the blending and denaturing of the proteins.

Store bought yogurt and kefir have denatured proteins, no enzymes, no vitamin B12, and just a few strains of bacteria added back to replace the multitudes that were destroyed. They are not short cuts, they are dead ends.

Wine

"Do not drink water any longer, but use a little wine for the sake of your stomach and your frequent cases of sickness," 1 Timothy 5:23. Sounds like medical advice to me. Since we will be using wine as medicine, we will want it to be as close as possible to the wine mentioned in 1st Timothy. This means the wine should be organic or biodynamic; in other words, without added sulfites, fungicides, or pesticides. Compared with conventional wine, organic red wines have been found to have up to 30% higher levels of polyphenols, such as reservatrol, and antioxidant activities. A growing body of research worldwide, on the benefits of wine, has prompted the World Health Organization (WHO), the US government, and the American Heart Association to issue statements highlighting scientific findings associating health benefits with the moderate use of wine. The fermentation process of turning grapes into wine gives us a powerful medicine from nature. Only a little wine is recommended, and that is all that is needed.

Apple Cider

You likely have never had apple cider made the traditional way, even though it was at one time the most popular beverage in the country and certainly one of the healthiest. In the late 1700s, an average citizen consumed more than 35 gallons of cider annually. Every estate, farm, and property had a few apple trees or an apple orchard. That was usually one of the first things a homesteader did, plant his apple trees. John Adams attributed his health and long life to a tankard of cider before breakfast. "From the founding of Jamestown, to the time of George Washington and Thomas Jefferson, on down to that of Robert E. Lee, every plantation owner made cider, drank cider, and bragged about his cider" (Hedrick, 1988).

What passes for cider today is only a faint caricature of the cider our founding forefathers drank. Like raw cheese and milk, forced pasteurization has turned a truly healthful beverage into a sweet drink of little benefit to the human body. So why, in the past, was cider considered safer than water to drink? Because it was fermented.

We searched and searched in the United States, the land once so proud of its cider, and could find none that were prepared completely the traditional way. Some were organic and did ferment the apples for the proper time, but they did so in stainless steel tanks, not the wooden barrels that our forefathers used. The wooden barrels are what create some of the health benefits of the apple cider. The apples react with the wood to create enzymes. We did find an online source from France, *Organic Etienne Dupont,* for apple cider fermented in wood. The apples are from their own ancient orchard. We don't expect most of you to order in apple cider, but it is easy to make. Since there is a short list of truly fermented foods available, we thought we would include it. As demand increases, maybe we won't have to go to France to get our cider.

APPLE CIDER VINEGAR

Apple cider vinegar is loaded with enzymes. If it agrees with you, then by all means, you should drink it. I would start with a little and work up; sip on it slowly. The apple cider you choose should be raw and organic. Bragg is a good brand. Just add ½ teaspoon of vinegar to a cup of warm, not hot, water.

Sauerkraut

Raw, organic, fermented sauerkraut will be vital to your recovery. Sauerkraut is thinly sliced cabbage which has been fermented. Its distinct sour flavor is the result of lacto-fermentation. Lactic acid, instead of vinegar, forms when bacteria in the fresh cabbage ferment the sugars. The art of preserving vegetables through fermentation goes back as far as 221 B.C., when it was discovered by the Chinese. Variants of fermented cabbage are used as food around the world.

Since neither refrigeration nor pasteurization is needed, the preservation of vegetables in this manner has provided man with a crucial source of nutrients in the winter for centuries. In fact, if the sauerkraut is pasteurized, all of the beneficial enzymes and lactic acid bacteria will be destroyed.

A healthy gut is very acidic and is populated with large numbers of beneficial bacteria. These bountiful, beneficial bacteria feed on the waste that remains from our digestion and create lactic acid. Our bodies depend on the lactic acid they produce to keep our gut healthy and in an acidic state. Without them, we would not have enough acidity to stop the growth of pathogenic parasites and yeasts. This can lead to an overgrowth of unfriendly yeasts, such as Candida albicans. Some of the symptoms of Candida yeast overgrowth are fatigue, intense food cravings, gas, poor memory, bad breath, and indigestion.

Lactobacilli plantarum is one of the beneficial strains of bacteria. It is found in only a few foods, but is abundant in sauerkraut. Lactobacilli plantarum is a dominant strain of probiotic bacteria that is known to actively aid in the digestive process. These strains of helpful bacteria also actively neutralize antinutrients, including phytic acid, which is found in grains, nuts, beans, etc.

The same beneficial bacteria that create lactic acid in the gut are naturally present in cabbage. They are what is responsible for turning raw cabbage into nutrient dense, highly digestible sauerkraut. The process of fermentation dramatically increases the number of these microorganisms as they digest the cabbage and produce lactic acid. When we ingest the sauerkraut, we replenish our gut with the beneficial bacteria that have been created. In addition, the lactic acid in the sauerkraut will enable the new bacteria to thrive, and in turn create more lactic acid in our guts.

The lactic acid in sauerkraut will also partially compensate for reduced hydrochloric acid in our stomachs. That is why it can have such a profound and immediate effect on digestive woes.

Raw sauerkraut is also a potent nutritional medicine. Due to its many anti-oxidant compounds, sauerkraut has strong anti-carcinogenic properties. The cancer fighting ability of raw sauerkraut was recently confirmed by the results from a nutritional study conducted at MTT Agrifood Research in Finland. The researchers made special note of the abundance of anti-oxidants, which are free radical scavengers useful in offsetting cellular damage that can lead to cancer. During the fermentation process, another nutrient, glucosinolate, is broken down by enzymes into powerful cancer fighting compounds called isothiocyanates. In addition, sauerkraut contains large amounts of certain antioxidants like lutein and zeaxanthin; both are associated with preserving ocular health. Sauerkraut is also known to have antibacterial and antiviral properties. In addition, sauerkraut contains many vital nutrients and essential minerals. Among them are calcium, potassium, and magnesium. Vitamin C is also found in abundance.

Perhaps most important of all for the fibromyalgia sufferer, unpasteurized sauerkraut is very high in viable enzymes that work just like the ones from the pancreas. In fact, the bacteria in sauerkraut (Lactobacillus plantarum) have been analyzed by DNA fingerprinting and shown to produce protease (Plengvidhya, 2007). For this reason, you should eat a little sauerkraut every time you consume protein.

In general, all fermented foods can be said to aid in the assimilation and digestion of proteins, but perhaps none better than raw sauerkraut. This will be your medicine, so it should not be mass produced and it needs to be organic (Bubbie's® is not organic).

We would like to share with you our favorite sauerkraut recipes. Enjoy!

Crocks and Crock Preparation for Sauerkraut Recipes

Ratios are based on a 5L crock. We use Harsch earthenware pickling crocks with a water reservoir. Harsch also makes a 7.5L and 10L crock that are good for home use. Many commercial sauerkraut purveyors have moved away from these old fashioned crocks and now use stainless steel or plastic. We believe, however, that these crocks are one of the reasons our sauerkraut is the best we have ever tasted.

To prepare your crock, first wash with a natural dish soap and then rinse thoroughly. You do not want to wash the crock with anything strong or harsh, as the crocks can take on the taste and odor. Also wash the crock weights in the dishwasher and then soak them in white vinegar. This method has prevented any mold or yeast formation in our sauerkraut.

Preparing Your Ingredients for Mixing

Wash the cabbage thoroughly. Peel off the outer leaves of the cabbage and reserve to place on top of the cabbage at the end of the process. Halve the cabbage and take out the core. Cut the cabbage into the thickness of a dime.

Chop up any other ingredients you want to add to give the sauerkraut flavor creating a veggie mixture. See our favorite recipes on pages 193 & 194.

Mixing Your Ingredients

Put one pound of cut cabbage in a bowl with 1 heaping teaspoon of sea salt. Using your hands, or a potato masher, work the sea salt into the cabbage to release the cell sap. Continue kneading until moist, but do not overwork. Overworking will make the cabbage limp and mushy.

Take a small handful of your veggie mixture and add to the pound of worked cabbage. Mix evenly.

Place the cabbage/veggie mixture into bottom of the crock. Repeat the above process in one pound increments, layering your cabbage/veggie mixture in the crock as you go. As you layer the ingredients press down to make sure cabbage/veggie mixture is tightly packed in the crock.

After Your Crock Is Full

When you have finished the layering process and reached the top, wipe down any excess cabbage from the sides and the top of the crock to prevent mold.

If the recipe calls for lemon or lime juice, pour the juice over the top of the cabbage in the crock.

Now layer the reserved outer leaves on top of the cabbage, so that none of it is exposed.

Place the crock weights on top of the cabbage and press down until the liquid rises above the stones. If the cabbage does not have a high enough moisture content to make the liquid rise above the stones, you will need to remove the stones and the cabbage leaves and add a salt-water solution or brine (33 oz of water to 2 tbsp of sea salt mixed until salt is dissolved). It is important to make sure that everything is submerged in the saltwater brine to preserve the cabbage as it ferments and to help prevent the formation of mold. Replace the outer cabbage leaves and stones. Wipe down any excess debris from the sides.

Put the lid on the crock and fill up the water well only half way. The water creates an air-tight barrier to prevent any dust, critters, etc. from getting into the sauerkraut.

Place the crock on two boards, or use something to elevate it, so that air can circulate under the crock. For the first 3 days, place the crock in an area of your home that is approximately 68-72 degrees. After three days, the temperature is less critical, but at that temperature it will take approximately three weeks to become sauerkraut. At cooler temperatures, the process may take three and a half to four weeks. You may see or hear air bubbles, which will let you know that the sauerkraut has begun fermenting.

You will periodically need to fill up the water well. Take care not to fill it so full that it gets into your sauerkraut.

After approximately three weeks, remove the lid, weights, and outer cabbage leaves carefully, so as not to contaminate the sauerkraut underneath. Place into jars and refrigerate. If the jars are unopened, the sauerkraut will last for 3-6 months. Once you begin opening the jar, it will last a week or two.

GARLIC LEMON DILL SAUERKRAUT

Ingredients:

- 1 large bunch of fresh organic dill. You may need to preorder at your health food store.
- 1 medium head of organic garlic
- 4.5 oz of Volcano® brand organic lemon juice (They come in 6.67oz lemon bursts or you can find it in large glass bottles).
- 9 lbs of organic green cabbage
- 3-4 outer leaves of the cabbage
- Celtic® sea salt

Preparation:

First, follow the instructions listed above in "Preparing Your Ingredients for Mixing." Then, wash dill, cut up, place in a bowl and set aside. Mince garlic and mix with dill so that the garlic and dill are mixed evenly.

Follow the instructions listed above in "Mixing Your Ingredients" and "After Your Crock Is Full."

SOUTH OF THE BORDER KRAUT

Recipe Courtesy of Christine Sanders

Ingredients (all organic):

- 9 pounds green cabbage
- 1 pound daikon radish
- 1 bunch red radishes
- 1 bunch green onions
- 2 bunches of cilantro
- ½ bulb of garlic
- 1 sweet onion
- ½ pound jalapenos (removing the seeds is optional to reduce the heat)

- 1 tsp each of coriander and celery seed
- 4.5 oz Volcano® brand lime burst and some fresh lime zest
- 1 tsp Celtic® sea salt per pound of cabbage

Preparation:

First, follow the instructions listed above in "Preparing Your Ingredients for Mixing." Then, mince the daikon radish, red radish, green onions, cilantro, garlic, sweet onion, and jalapenos. Mix all these ingredients together evenly. Add the coriander, celery seed, and lime zest to the vegetable mix, mix evenly, and place in a separate bowl.

Follow the instructions listed above in "Mixing Your Ingredients" and "After Your Crock Is Full."

BEET, CARROT, GINGER KRAUT

Recipe Courtesy of Christine Sanders

Ingredients (all organic):

- 9 pounds of green cabbage
- 4 medium red beets
- 4 large carrots (shredded)
- 1 bunch green onion
- 2-3 inch of ginger root (peeled and minced fine)
- 1/2 small bulb garlic (cloves peeled and minced)
- 1 small bunch dill
- 1 tsp Celtic® sea salt per pound of cabbage

Preparation:

First, follow the instructions listed above in "Preparing Your Ingredients for Mixing." Then, wash and cut up the beets, green onions, and dill. Add shredded carrots, minced ginger, and minced garlic. Mix all these ingredients together evenly and place in a separate bowl.

Follow the instructions listed above in "Mixing Your Ingredients" and "After Your Crock Is Full."

RAW FERMENTED SWEET PICKLE RELISH

We love this recipe because it is delicious and a great way to get another fermented food in your diet without any special equipment.

Ingredients:

- 1 organic cucumber
- ½ organic small red or green bell pepper
- ½ teaspoon sea salt

Preparation:

Shred the veggies with a grater, food processor, or dice them finely. Put them in a jar with ½ teaspoon salt. Cap loosely or cover with cheesecloth and a rubber band and store in a cool dry place for three days or more. The warmer the storage place, the shorter the fermenting time. The texture should be crisp and the taste should be salty, sweet, and tangy. Replace the lid and refrigerate in between uses.

BEET KVASS

A sweet and salty lacto-fermented beverage infused with all of the vitamins, minerals, and detoxifying properties of beets.

Ingredients:

- 5 large organic beets (any variety).
- 2 tablespoons sea salt finely ground.

Preparation

1. Peel the beets. Chop them into one-inch cubes.
2. Combine the sea salt and the chopped beets and place the mixture in a half-gallon jar.
3. Add enough water to fill the jar (well, spring, or filtered water is best), leaving about two-inches of space at the top. Stir to

dissolve the salt and cover with a cloth or paper towel secured by a rubber band.

4. Allow to ferment in a warm spot of your kitchen for about 2 days before moving it to the refrigerator.

BONE BROTHS

Science has confirmed what Grandma always knew, that broth made from bones is not just soup, but medicine. Bone broth, used throughout history, has been affectionately called "Jewish penicillin." It contains highly absorbable forms of calcium, magnesium, potassium, phosphorous, and sulfur, as well as trace minerals.

Bone broth is very soothing and healing to the gut. One of its main constituents is gelatin. Gelatin is a lubricating substance that coats and protects the mucous membranes of the gut. Since bone broth is soothing and highly nutritious, it will help restore your gut to health.

Store bought, canned soup will not do. You will need to make it the way Grandma did. You can simmer a big batch and freeze it for many meals to come. It really is not difficult or time consuming to make. My favorite bone broth is chicken and rice.

Here is the recipe:

CHICKEN AND RICE SOUP

Ingredients:

- 1 whole organic pastured chicken
- 2 large organic carrots
- 2 organic celery ribs
- 1 quartered organic onion
- 6 cloves organic garlic peeled and smashed
- 2 cups cooked organic brown rice (soak the rice 1-2 hours before cooking to remove the phytic acid)
- 1 organic bay leaf
- sea salt and pepper to taste

Preparation:

Wash the chicken well and put it in a large stock pot. Cover with water. Chop the carrots and celery into large chunks, quarter the onion and add to stock pot. Add garlic. Season with salt, pepper, and a bay leaf. Simmer for 2 hours or until chicken is tender.

Remove carrots, celery, and onion. Chop up the carrots into small chunks and add back to soup. Remove chicken, shred or dice, and add back to soup. Add 2 cups of cooked brown rice. That's it, you're done!

SLOW COOKER CHICKEN BONE BROTH

Ingredients:

- 1 whole organic grass-fed chicken frame (leftover bones from a roasted chicken)
- 1 quartered organic onion
- 7 cloves of organic garlic peeled and smashed
- 1 organic bay leaf
- sea salt and pepper to taste

Preparation:

Place all of your ingredients in your slow cooker, cover with cold filtered water and turn on low.

Allow to cook on low for 12 hours and then you can begin using the broth. As you remove broth from your slow cooker, replace that amount with cold-filtered water.

Pour the broth through a fine strainer to remove solids and drink.

Continue to cook on low for up to 24 hours.

After 24 hours remove the remaining broth and discard the chicken bones. To store any remaining broth, allow to cool and place in glass containers. The broth will last in the refrigerator for several days or several months in the freezer.

GARLIC BEEF BONE BROTH

Ingredients:

- 4 lbs of beef bones from organic pastured cows
- 2 organic roughly chopped medium carrots
- 2 organic roughly chopped medium celery stalks
- 1 organic chopped medium onion
- 8 organic garlic cloves, peeled and smashed
- 2 organic bay leaves
- ½ teaspoon sea salt
- 2 tablespoons of organic apple cider vinegar
- cold filtered water

Preparation:

Put the bones in a stockpot and cover with water. Bring to a boil and remove any foam that rises to the surface, while leaving the floating fat. Once it reaches a boil turn down to a simmer.

Add the vegetables, garlic, bay leaves, sea salt, and vinegar.

Cover and simmer for 12 hours-48 hours. The longer you cook the stock, the more rich, flavorful, and medicinal it will be.

When it is finished, remove the bones and pour the broth through a strainer, discarding the solids. If the broth is overly greasy from the fat on the bones, refrigerate the broth overnight and then remove the white fat layer on top.

Store the finished broth in glass containers. Allow to cool completely before refrigerating or freezing. The broth will last in the refrigerator for several days or several months in the freezer.

When ready to drink, gently heat the broth on the stove until liquid.

FOODS RICH IN VITAMIN B12

If you have a profound deficiency in vitamin B12, then you will need to eat proteins, at least temporarily, that contain very high levels of B12. The recommended dietary allowance (RDA) for vitamin B12 is 2.4 mcg. One chicken breast, one egg, and a cup of yogurt, for example, would need to be consumed daily just to meet the day's minimum requirement. There would be nothing left to make up the deficit that led to many of the symptoms associated with fibromyalgia.

Clams, oysters, and mussels all contain very high levels of B12. Clams provide the most with 98.9 mcg per 100 g serving. For a 3 oz serving, that would be 1401% of the RDA. Just one small clam would give you 156.6% of the RDA. If you make a big pot of clam chowder and freeze it in small shot-glass size containers, you could have an appetizer serving daily that would boost your B12 levels immensely. Just make sure to source your clams carefully. Sorry, canned clams won't do, as they contain high levels of bisphenol-A (BPA), a known endocrine disruptor that has been linked to cardiovascular disease, diabetes, obesity, and liver abnormalities.

Bisphenol-A is used to make polycarbonate plastic bottles and epoxy can linings. We have all heard about the dangers of plastic bottles, but a new study by researchers at Harvard School of Public Health found that people who ate just 12 ounces of canned soup for only 5 days had a 1,221% greater concentration of BPA in their urine (Carwile, 2011). The study's lead author stated that, "This study suggests that canned foods may be an even greater concern (than plastic bottles), especially given their wider use." Research has also shown that bisphenol-A disrupts the kynurenine pathway, which would have direct implications for someone with fibromyalgia (Zasshi, 2004).

Next on the list would be organic pastured liver. The liver of almost any animal is loaded with B12 (B12 is stored in the liver). Lamb, beef, duck, and goose liver are all good choices. Lamb liver provides 72.85 mcg (230% RDA) in a 3 oz serving.

Caviar, octopus, fish, crab, and lobster all contain high amounts of B12, but are not in the same category as clams, oysters, mussels, and liver. The proteins that most of us consume, such as beef, chicken, cheese, and eggs do have B12, and we will benefit by eating them, but an egg, for instance, has just 0.33 mcg per yolk or only 6% of the RDA.

No matter what protein you choose, the most important thing to remember is to consume it with a fermented vegetable, such as sauerkraut. Here is a recipe for our favorite clam (or oyster) chowder. Make a big pot and freeze some for many meals to come.

CLAM CHOWDER

Ingredients (all organic):

- 1 quart shucked clams
- 1/3 pound salt pork
- 1 large white or yellow onion, minced
- 2 celery stalks, minced
- 2 large baking potatoes, diced
- 1 bay leaf
- ½ teaspoon thyme
- 1 quart raw milk
- ½ cup unsalted butter (pastured raw butter is best), melted
- 1 cup all-purpose flour or, even better, 1 cup whole-wheat flour
- coarse sea-salt
- fresh ground white or black pepper

Preparation:

- Drain and chop clams, reserving liquid.
- In a heavy pan, fry the salt pork until all fat is rendered.
- Toss in the onions and celery and brown lightly.
- Add the butter and flour and stir constantly for 5 minutes.
- Add potatoes, clam liquid, bay leaf, and thyme.
- Simmer the soup until potatoes are fork tender.
- Add chopped clams and milk.
- Simmer 3-5 minutes.
- Allow to cool and freeze in glass containers.

Green Smoothies

Green smoothies are a delicious way to provide your body with much needed enzymes and many other healthful nutrients as well. They also provide a good nutritional return for the small amount of time and energy required to prepare them. Here are two of our favorite green smoothie recipes:

TANGERINE GINGER GREEN SMOOTHIE

Ingredients (all organic):

- 2 slices of fresh ginger root
- 1 kiwi
- 1 tangerine
- 1 apple
- 1 handful baby spinach

Preparation:

Put all ingredients into blender. Fill with cold water 3/4 of the way up the blender. Blend and pour into a chilled glass. Enjoy!

BANANA MANGO GREEN SMOOTHIE

Ingredients (all organic):

- 1 cup mango or papaya
- 1/2 cup kale
- 1/2 cup spinach
- 1/2 banana
- 1/2 green apple

Preparation:

Put all ingredients into blender. Blend until smooth. Enjoy!

NUTS AND SEEDS

Nuts and seeds are a precious source of nutrition. They are brimming with enzymes. However, there is a caveat, you need to soak them. I know, that sounded strange to me too at first. Nuts and seeds naturally contain large amounts of enzyme inhibitors to keep them from sprouting before their appointed time.

In nature, the growth cycle is triggered by rain. Nuts and seeds are waiting for this signal. The rain washes off the enzyme inhibitors, so it can germinate and grow into a plant. Soaking the nuts and seeds mimics this natural signal and washes away the enzyme inhibitors. This allows your body to benefit from all the vitamins and enzymes within the nuts and seeds. Nuts and seeds that are not soaked are very difficult to digest and will actually deplete your body's store of existing enzymes.

Soaking nuts and seeds was done by the people who came before us. It is the traditional method of preparation. The Aztecs would soak pumpkin and squash seeds in salt water and then dry them in the sun. This is still done today in parts of Central America. Since we are trying to restore enzymes and want to benefit from the wonderful store of nutrients and enzymes that nuts and seeds have to offer, we will want to soak them too.

One would think that soaking nuts and seeds would rob them of their flavor and crisp texture, but just the opposite is true. Soaking nuts and seeds actually improves their taste and texture.

The process of soaking nuts and seeds simply involves soaking them in warm salt water for a period of time and then drying them. The nuts or seeds do need to be thoroughly dried or they could become moldy and they should not be dried at temperatures higher than 150 °F. Higher temperatures will destroy beneficial enzymes. The nuts or seeds can be dried in a food dehydrator or an oven. If your oven doesn't go below 200 °F, you can set the oven to the lowest temperature and leave the door slightly ajar. After soaking and drying, the nuts or seeds can be stored in the refrigerator for a few days.

The following recipe for soaked almonds is from the cookbook Nourishing Traditions by Sally Fallon. We do recommend using organic nuts.

SOAKED ALMONDS

Ingredients:

- 4 cups almonds (insecticide free is best)
- 1 tablespoon sea salt
- filtered water

Preparation:

Mix almonds with salt and cover with filtered water. Leave in a warm place for at least 7 hours or overnight. Drain in a colander. Spread on a stainless steel baking pan and place in a warm oven for around 24 hours (no more than 150 °F or 65 °C as this will kill the enzymes). Stir occasionally, until completely dry and crisp. Store in an air-tight container.

Skinless almonds will still sprout, indicating that the process of removing their skins has not destroyed the enzymes. Skinless almonds are easier to digest and more satisfactory in many recipes. However, you may also use almonds with skins on. You can use slivered almond pieces for this recipe.

You can also crisp peanuts, pine nuts, hazelnuts, macadamia nuts, cashews (as the enzymes in cashews are destroyed when they are processed it is best to roast quickly and soak no more than 6 hours). Makes 4 cups.

Raw Honey

Raw honey is a food noted for its exceptionally high enzyme content. "Raw" means that it has not been heated to the point where all the beneficial enzymes have been killed. The enzymes in raw honey help to initiate the process of digestion and reduce the body's need to produce digestive enzymes. Due to its high enzyme content, raw honey spares the enzyme reserves of the pancreas and other digestive organs. Raw honey also has many other health benefits. It helps with seasonal allergies, is antibacterial, boosts the immune system, and combats yeast overgrowth in the body.

Raw, organic honey should become your new sweetener. You can use it on your oatmeal in the morning, in your kefir smoothies, and for virtually anything else in which you would use sugar.

It is extremely important to avoid the use of all artificial sweeteners, such as aspartame. Aspartame, also known as NutraSweet or Equal, can be found in a variety of food products including soft drinks, yogurt, puddings, frozen desserts, baked goods, chewing gum and other candies. One study found that aspartame significantly reduced *glutathione* and substantially increased *tumor necrosis factor* (Abdel-Salam, 2012). It also caused a dose-dependent inhibition of *serotonin, noradrenaline, and dopamine*. No wonder there have been reports of it being associated with fibromyalgia (Ciappuccini, 2010).

Making sure your honey is raw and organic is vital though, because not all honey is created equal. Many harmful chemicals can be used in producing non-organic honey. In addition, some honey producers are either feeding their bees corn syrup or adding corn syrup to the honey to increase profits. So, raw, organic honey is the only honey that you should be eating.

We have provided a great source for raw honey in the resource section of this book, but you can also find wonderful local raw honey by visiting farmers' markets and using sources such as www.localharvest.org.

GIVE UP THE SUGAR (AND ARTIFICIAL SWEETENERS), BUT NOT THE CHOCOLATE!

The antioxidant benefits of dark chocolate have long been known, but research now shows that raw cocoa directly feeds the beneficial bacteria in your gastrointestinal (GI) tract. In addition to increased levels of beneficial bacteria, a preliminary clinical trial also observed an accompanying decrease in bacteria associated with diarrhea and constipation. Raw cocoa also decreased blood levels of triglycerides, cholesterol, and C-Reactive protein (a marker of inflammation associated with heart disease).

Cacao beans go through a fermentation process, so this might help explain their positive effect on bacterial levels in our guts. If you drink a cup of hot chocolate made with enzyme rich honey, gut boosting cocoa powder, and raw milk, you will have a truly enjoyable way of replenishing your GI tract.

HONEY HOT CHOCOLATE

Ingredients:

- 1 tablespoon raw honey
- 1 tablespoon organic raw cocoa
- 1 cup of organic raw milk

Preparation:

Mix together honey and cocoa into a paste. Add paste to the milk and heat slowly and gently on the stove until just hot. Do not allow to boil, as we want to keep as many beneficial bacteria and enzymes as we can. Add more honey and cocoa to taste. You can also make delicious chocolate milk with this recipe.

CHOCOLATE CHAI

We love this recipe! It is hot chocolate for adults.

Ingredients:

- ¼ cup water
- 1 organic black tea bag (be sure to use an unbleached tea bag with a string or loose leaf tea)
- 1 1/2 tablespoons raw honey
- 2 tablespoons organic unsweetened cocoa powder
- 2 cups organic raw milk
- 1 teaspoon organic vanilla extract
- ½ teaspoon organic ground cinnamon

- ½ teaspoon organic ground nutmeg
- sweetened whip cream (see recipe below)
- 2 (3 inch) organic cinnamon sticks (optional)

Preparation:

1. Bring the water to a boil in a small saucepan. Add the tea bag, cover, and remove from the heat. Let stand for 3 to 5 minutes.
2. Remove the tea bag and stir in the honey and cocoa. Return to the stove over medium heat and bring just to a boil.
3. Mix in the milk, vanilla, cinnamon and nutmeg, heat through but do not boil.
4. Pour into mugs and top with whipped cream and a cinnamon stick garnish.

Makes 2 servings

SWEETENED WHIP CREAM

Ingredients:

- 1/2 cup fresh raw cream
- 1 1/2 teaspoons raw honey
- Dash of organic vanilla extract

Preparation:

Put all ingredients in a chilled glass or stainless steel bowl and mix with an electric mixer until peaks form.

FRUIT AND HONEY FERMENTED SODA

This lacto-fermented "pop" is one of the most enjoyable ways to ingest beneficial bacteria and enzymes. It is actually good for you!

Ingredients and Preparation:

Starter

- Add 1 tablespoon fresh organic grated ginger and 2 teaspoons raw honey to 1 quart cold water. Stir together. Cover with cheesecloth or an unbleached paper towel and secure with metal lid ring or a rubber band.

- Place on a cool part of the counter.
- Every day add 2 teaspoons of ginger and 2 teaspoons of honey and stir.
- After one week, cover with an air-tight lid. Place in the refrigerator.

Pop

- 6 cups of organic fruit (strawberries, blueberries, rhubarb, etc. depending on what you want the flavor of the pop to be)
- 1 cup of raw organic honey
- 2 quarts cold water
- 1 cup of starter (see above)

Add fruit, honey, and cold water to pan. Warm just enough to dissolve the honey. Once honey is dissolved, allow mixture to cool and pour into a gallon jar and add 1 cup of pop starter.

Note: Do not add starter if mixture is too hot, as this will kill the live bacteria. Let cool until lukewarm.

Cover jar with cheesecloth or an unbleached paper towel. Let sit on the counter for one to three days. Taste on first day and if the pop doesn't have enough fizz, let it go another day or so. The longer the pop ferments, the less sweet it will be. Strain into a clean jar and cover with an airtight lid.

Refrigerate and enjoy!

CHAPTER 27

Medicinal Teas

Block Tumor Necrosis Factor Naturally (and deliciously)

A relative of ginger, turmeric is a powder ground from the root of a large-leafed Asian plant. Turmeric is a potent antioxidant. Research shows that turmeric is also a powerful blocker of tumor necrosis factor.

"The active component of turmeric turns out to be the best blocker yet of a natural chemical called TNF, or tumor necrosis factor, which contributes to cancers and arthritis and is resistant to chemotherapy drugs," stated Bharat B. Aggarwal, professor of cancer medicine in the Department of Experimental Therapeutics at the University of Texas M.D. Anderson Cancer Center, who has studied the spice for a decade. "You don't even need tens of thousands of dollars of TNF blockers," Aggarwal stated. "Turmeric does exactly the same thing."

The benefits of naturally controlling tumor necrosis factor for a patient with fibromyalgia would be immense. Not only would the conditions that result directly from elevated tumor necrosis factor be resolved, but the rapid degradation of tryptophan through the kynurenine pathway would be halted as well. Symptoms such as IBS, depression, anxiety, inflammation of the fascia, etc. would be directly addressed through this amazing spice.

Traditionally, turmeric has been consumed with some type of fat. In a typical curry, for example, turmeric root will be cooked in oil. Some of the ancient Ayurvedic texts recommend cooking turmeric in fatty buffalo milk. This ancient wisdom serves us well today. Turmeric is not absorbed well by the body unless it is consumed with some fat. Turmeric tea made with raw goat or cow's milk will help your body properly absorb turmeric. It would be beneficial to consume 1-2 cups throughout the day.

TURMERIC TEA

Ingredients (all organic):

- 1 cup raw milk (goat's or cow's)
- 1/2 teaspoon turmeric
- 1 teaspoon cinnamon
- 1/4 teaspoon ginger
- 1 teaspoon raw honey or to taste

Preparation:

Heat the milk on the stovetop until hot, stir in the spices and drizzle the honey on top. Stir and enjoy!

GARLIC LOWERS HOMOCYSTEINE

Research has shown that garlic can have a profound effect on homocysteine (Yeh, 2006). Dr. Matthew Budoff, M.D., Professor of Medicine at UCLA states, "Studies have shown that garlic supplementation can lower homocysteine levels by up to 35%." Many of the disease conditions caused by elevated levels of homocysteine in fibromyalgia, such as migraines, mitral valve prolapse, hypermobility, low magnesium, endometriosis, and increased risk of cancer could be dramatically reduced by daily ingestion of garlic.

Garlic can be ingested in a variety of ways. For instance, it can be added to bone broths to increase their medicinal value, as we have done in our bone broth recipes. Look for other recipes and opportunities in your daily cooking to include garlic. Garlic can also be taken in capsule form. Just be sure it is pure organic whole garlic, not an extract. Garlic tea is also a very beneficial way to consume garlic.

The following recipe for garlic tea came from a friend's mother who is a native of Mexico. Garlic tea is a favorite home remedy in Mexico and Spain due to its additional healthful properties of being a potent antibacterial and antiviral. When using garlic tea to fight a bacterial or viral infection, we find it is especially effective if you start drinking it at the first sign of illness and continue drinking until you are fully recovered. You can double the recipe and drink throughout the course of the day.

GARLIC TEA

Ingredients:

- 3–4 cloves organic garlic, smashed with a knife
- 3–4 cups of water
- Raw honey to taste
- Fresh squeezed organic lemon juice to taste

Preparation:

Place smashed cloves of garlic and water in a saucepan and heat to a gentle simmer. Reduce heat slightly and let steep with the lid on until the tea has achieved a strong garlic taste. Add honey and lemon to taste.

Chamomile Tea

I rarely drink plain water. As I write this, it is 10:00 p.m. on the dot and I am enjoying a cup of chamomile tea. Of course, it has water in it, but it is boosted with the health benefits of this powerful, but gentle herb. Chamomile tea should be on your beverage list for many reasons. It contains compounds that will soothe and heal a damaged GI tract. It is a wonderful sleep aid, due to its calming and relaxing properties. It also reduces inflammation, relieves muscle spasms, and has antiviral and antibacterial benefits.

Recently, research has shown chamomile to be effective in fighting diabetes. In one study, after 21 days, diabetic rats that received chamomile had significantly lower blood glucose levels than rats that did not.

To make my tea though, I didn't just open a box, put a tea bag in hot water, and call it a day. Here's why. Often, to get the tea in the bag, the herb is nearly powdered. This creates fissures, or cuts, on the surface of the herb. This is also true of other herbs in tea bags. These fissures immediately start to oxidize because they are now exposed to the air. They begin to lose flavor and beneficial health properties. When you are using an herb for its medicinal properties, it should be as fresh and potent as possible. To reap all of the benefits tea has to offer, I use organic loose leaf tea and brew it in a tea pot with a strainer. Remember, they are just foods. You wouldn't shred an apple weeks or months before you were ready to eat it, would you?

There is another, and perhaps even greater, concern. Does your tea bag look like a white pillow? Is it bright white with no string stapled to it? Then it has most likely been heat sealed with a potent carcinogen called polyvinyl chloride. It is white because it has been bleached with another potent carcinogen called dioxin. Both of these chemicals are heat released and water soluble. Do you know what that means? When you add this bag to a cup of hot water, you are drinking two of the most dangerous chemicals on this planet.

I ordered some bath herbs once from an herbalist who had taken great care in the growing and harvesting of the herbs, so I was quite surprised when I received them and they were in the pillow tea bags. I called and asked her if she had used polyvinyl chloride to seal them and explained my concern. Even though I wasn't drinking it, I didn't want to take a bath in it either. She said, "It's funny you say that, I used my iron to seal them, and it gunked the iron up so badly, I can't use it for anything else!"

If you use tea bags at all, be sure they have a drawstring and the bag is not bleached white. It costs the tea company a fraction of a cent more to do it this way, but I am grateful they value our well-being enough to do this.

I rarely drink tea made with tea bags, simply because it doesn't come close in quality and flavor to a tea made from the whole herb. Once you know how to do it, it is the simplest thing in the world.

CHAMOMILE TEA

Instructions:

- Bring 2 cups of water just to the boiling point
- Put 3 tablespoons organic whole chamomile flower (loose leaf tea) in a 2 cup tea pot
- Add hot water and steep for 10 minutes or until desired strength
- Strain (add honey if desired) and enjoy

Green Tea

There are many health benefits associated with drinking green tea. The antioxidants in green tea have been found to be over 100 times more effective in neutralizing free radicals than vitamin C and 25 times more powerful than vitamin E. These same antioxidants have been found to reduce cellular damage that could lead to cancer.

Like chamomile, green tea is also noted for its anti-viral and anti-bacterial properties, which would assist protease and the immune system in their ongoing battle to keep the body free from viruses and pathogenic bacteria.

Another amazing property of green tea is that it is calming, and yet energizing at the same time. Only nature could accomplish that. The calming effects of green tea are due to a compound called L-theanine. Research has shown that L-theanine increases GABA levels. Numerous benefits would be associated with increased levels of GABA for the fibromyalgia sufferer.

GREEN TEA

Instructions:

- Bring 2 cups of water almost to the boiling point
- Add 2 tablespoons loose organic green tea leaves to a 2 cup tea pot
- Steep for 2 minutes and taste for desired strength
- Strain and enjoy!

Black Tea

I love the full and rich flavor of black tea. Black tea actually undergoes a fermentation process of its own. Researchers are learning that the health benefits of black tea are just as numerous as green tea. It is full of anti-oxidants, can block DNA damage, and help the body detoxify harmful chemicals. By adding raw cream and honey, it has taken the place of the sugary pick me up I used to reach for in the afternoon when my energy would dip.

BLACK TEA

Instructions:

- Bring 2 cups of water just to the boiling point
- Add 3 tablespoons organic loose leaf black tea leaves
- Steep for 4-5 minutes to desired strength.
- Strain, add raw cream and honey to taste. Enjoy!

Herbal Bitters

Bitter herbs, such as chamomile, hops, dandelion, yarrow, and more, have been used for centuries as a digestive aid and are still a part of many traditional cultures all over the world. Herbal bitters are named for these bitter tasting plants they are derived from.

Herbal bitters work by preparing your body to digest the food you are about to eat. As soon as they touch your taste buds, they stimulate the stomach, liver, gallbladder, and pancreas to begin secreting substances such as gastric juices, bile, and insulin. They work when taken as an aperitif, digestive aid, or to settle an upset stomach. Instead of interfering with the digestive process, like many antacid medications, they work to support it.

CHAPTER 28

Sample Daily Menu

THIS IS A SAMPLE MENU of what a typical day's diet should look like. Your emphasis should be on foods that heal the digestive tract and supply the body with essential missing nutrients, such as vitamin B12. Always be sure to consume a raw fermented vegetable, such as sauerkraut, every time you eat an animal protein. There is no need to limit your portions with these deeply healing and nutritious foods. Let your own body guide you in the portions you require.

SAMPLE DAILY MENU

Breakfast:

- Bowl of soaked organic oatmeal topped with organic fruit, raw organic milk, and honey or maple syrup to taste
- Kefir smoothie made with organic fruit and raw organic honey. We make a double batch and drink one or two cups throughout the day.
- Organic coffee, hot chocolate, green, black, or herbal tea

Snack:

- Raw organic pastured cheese with whole grain sourdough bread or crackers

Lunch:

- Bone Broth
- ¼ to ½ cup sauerkraut or other raw organic fermented vegetable

- Pastured organic turkey, chicken, or egg salad sandwich on sourdough bread

Snack:

- Green smoothie
- 1/3 cup soaked organic nuts or seeds

Dinner:

- Clam chowder
- Whole grain sourdough bread with raw organic pastured butter or organic olive oil
- ¼ to ½ cup raw organic fermented sauerkraut or other fermented vegetable

Snacks:

- Turmeric tea
- Fresh organic fruit

Remember this isn't a "diet," this is a healthy new way of eating. The point is not to go hungry or starve yourself, it is to fill your body with nutrient dense foods that will heal your digestive tract and help you recover.

Your diet should be reminiscent of foods that would have been eaten on a family farm 100 years ago. Copious amounts of garden fresh vegetables in the summer and raw fermented vegetables in the winter, squashes and potatoes from the root cellar, raw milk, cream and cheese, pastured eggs and meats, wild game, organ meats (such as liver), whole grains, sourdough bread, berries, apples, and other fresh fruits in season were all daily fare.

Here is a list of whole food blog sites that are packed with recipes for traditional foods. You can customize your diet based on your time, energy, and resources.

http://www.realfoodforlessmoney.com/
http://www.passionatehomemaking.com/

http://www.culturesforhealth.com/
http://www.pantryparatus.com/
http://www.holisticsquid.com/
http://nourishedkitchen.com/
http://www.gnowflins.com/
http://www.cookingtf.com
http://www.thehealthyhomeeconomist.com/
http://ohlardy.com/

CHAPTER 29

The Best Way to Eliminate Harmful Pathogens: Set a Mousetrap

IN ORDER TO COMPLETELY HEAL your GI tract and restore your body's ability to properly digest proteins and other nutrients, you will need to address the small intestine bacterial overgrowth (SIBO) found in patients with fibromyalgia. Most likely, there is also an overgrowth of pathogenic yeasts as well. The use of a conventional antibiotic or antifungal, though, will just further damage your GI tract. We need to protect our beneficial bacteria and enzymes while we destroy the pathogenic organisms. Nature has provided us with something to do just that – antibacterial and antifungal herbs.

When you have a mouse in the house, I think it is far better to set a mousetrap than to blow up the entire house to catch it. Herbs are the mousetrap. They will do the job of conventional antibiotics and antifungals without causing damage to your 'house'.

Golden seal, myrrh, garlic, echinacea, and slippery elm are some common and extremely effective antibacterial and antifungal herbs. These herbs are just whole foods and your body will recognize and benefit from them in many ways. Instead of having "side effects", they have what we like to call "side benefits". Garlic, for instance, in addition to being a potent antibacterial and anti-viral, also lowers homocysteine.

These herbs should be organic or wild crafted and in their whole form. We have our own blend of antibacterial and antifungal capsules available on our website-www.naturehaditfirst.com.

CHAPTER 30

Your Future

I PROMISE, YOU HAVE NEVER HAD FOOD LIKE THIS. Your body most likely has never been truly nourished. Growing up, a typical school day lunch for me was a bologna sandwich on white bread and a Twinkie®. So, I know how foreign this new diet must sound. But when you start to eat living foods, your body will come alive too. It will also simplify your life. These foods are so satisfying, on such a deep level, that you won't crave processed food. Your brain won't constantly be sensing that your body hasn't been nourished, and subsequently keep driving you to eat more in order to find real nutrition. You will lose weight, you will lower your cholesterol, your blood sugars will normalize, your blood pressure will go down, and your energy will go up.

Nature gave us sauerkraut for winter, since we wouldn't have the fruit from fall trees or carrots from the summer gardens. Nature gave us cucumbers in the summer to be turned into pickles for the winter, so we would always have vital bacteria and enzymes. These are special foods. Nature has set them aside. They are unique in every way. Nothing can replace them; nothing else will do.

CHAPTER 31

Resources

OUR RESOURCES ARE NOT 'BIG BUSINESS', but rather small proprietors that are artisans of their craft. We know many of them personally and have spoken to them at length about how they make their products. We are sharing with you the foods that are at our own dinner tables. Enjoy!

SAUERKRAUT, PICKLES, AND OTHER VEGETABLES

Kaptain's Kraut- Lemon Garlic Dill Sauerkraut—
This is our favorite sauerkraut!
(425)443-7079

Happy Girl Kitchen Co.- canned tomatoes (in glass jars), classic dill pickles, and summer jam
www.HappyGirlKitchen.com/

Real Pickles- sauerkraut and pickles
www.RealPickles.com

Cultured Pickle Shop- sauerkraut
www.CulturedPickleShop.com
(510)540-5185

Thirty AcreFarm- sauerkraut, Kim chi, and real pickles
www.ThirtyAcreFarm.com

MILK, KEFIR, AND CHEESE

Raw Milk- find resources in your area
www.RealMilk.com

Raw Cheese- organic, pastured cheese
www.JamesRanch.net

Kefir Grains- grains, jars and instructions
www.NatureHadItFirst.com or www.Etsy.com

BEEF, CHICKEN, PORK, AND SHELLFISH

Good Earth Farms- organic, pastured beef, chicken, and pork
www.GoodEarthFarms.com

Kachemak Shellfish Growers-for oysters grown in the pristine glacier-fed waters of Alaska
http://alaskaoyster.com/cm/

Dorsey Creek Organics-a wonderful family source for organic beef cattle, hogs, dairy cows, eggs, oats, spelt, rye, wheat, barley, corn, alfalfa seed, clover seed, and vegetable crops including rhubarb and asparagus.
http://www.dorseycreekorganics.com
stanjones53@hotmail.com or (307)-250-4325

Vital Choice Seafood-wild caught salmon, shellfish, berries and much more.
www.vitalsource.com

OTHER WONDERFUL FINDS

Living Nutz- organic germinated nuts
www.LivingNutz.com

Healing Spirits Herb Farm- one of the best herbalists in the country, and my mentor, Andrea Reisen.
www.HealingSpiritsHerbFarm.com (607)566-2701

Tropical Traditions- honey and organic coconut oil
www.TropicalTraditions.com

Northwest Wild Foods-wild blueberries, blackberries, huckleberries and more, perfect for your kefir smoothie or on your morning muesli.
http://www.nwwildfoods.com

Books and Resources

Nourishing Traditions by Sally Fallon

The Idiot's Guide to Fermentation by Wardeh Harmon

Wild Fermentation by Sandor Katz

The Raw Family for more information on green smoothies and delicious recipes.
www.RawFamily.com

Environmental Working Group to find the toxicity rating of the beauty and bath products we use on our skin every day.
http://www.ewg.org/skindeep/

Eat Wild for information on where to find grass-fed foods in your area.
www.EatWild.com

Local Harvest is a great website to find many locally raised foods, including farmer's markets and CSA programs.
www.LocalHarvest.org

REFERENCES

Abdel-Salam, O.M., N.A. Salem, J.S. Hussein. 2012. Effect of aspartame on oxidative stress and monoamine neurotransmitter levels in lipopolysaccharide-treated mice. *Neurotox Res.* 21(3):245-55. doi: 10.1007/s12640-011-9264-9. Epub 2011 Aug 6.

Alsfasser G., B. Antoniu, S.P. Thayer, A.L. Warshaw, C. Fernández-del Castillo. 2005. Degradation and inactivation of plasma tumor nec osis factor-alpha by pancreatic proteases in experimental acute pancreatitis. *Pancreatology* 5(1):37-43.

American Heritage Dictionary. 2003. Definition of Arsenic. Retrieved on 1/21/2013 from http://ahdictionary.com/word/search.html?q=arsenic&submit.x=0&submit.y=0.

Amital, D., C. Herskovitz, L. Fostick, A. Silberman, Y. Doron, J. Zohar, A. Itsekson, M. Zolti, A. Rubinow, H. Amital. 2004. The Premenstrual Syndrome and Fibromyalgia. *Clinical Reviews in Allergy and Immunology* Volume 38, Issue 2-3, pp 107-115.

Allen, R. 2004. Dopamine and iron in the pathophysiology of restless legs syndrome (RLS). *Sleep Med* 5(4):385-91.

Armstrong, D.J., G.K. Meenagh, I. Bickle, A.S. Lee, E.S. Curran, M.B. Finch. 2007. Vitamin D deficiency is associated with anxiety and depression in fibromyalgia. *Clin Rheumatol.* (4):551-4. Epub 2006 Jul 19.

Arthritis Today. 2009. *What is Fibromyalgia?* ArthritisToday.org. Retrieved 6/9/2011 from http:// www.arthritistoday.org/conditions/fibromyalgia/all-about-fibro/what-is-fibromyalgia.php

Bagge, E., B.A. Bengtsson, L. Carlsson, J. Carlsson. 1998. Low growth hormone secretion in patients with fibromyalgia--a preliminary report on 10 patients and 10 controls. *J Rheumatol.* 25(1):145-8.

Bakowski, M. 1999. Pancreatic enzymes and fibrosing colonopathy. *Lancet* Jul 17;354(9174):249.

Baraniuk, J.N., B. Casado, H. Maibach, D.J. Clauw, L.K. Pannell, S. Hess. 2005. A chronic fatigue syndrome-related proteome in human cerebrospinal fluid. *BMC Neurol* 5:22. Published online 2005 December 1. doi: 10.1186/1471-2377-5-22 PMCID: PMC1326206.

Bazzichi, L., L. Palego, G. Giannaccini, A. Rossi, F. De Feo, C. Giacomelli, L. Betti, L. Giusti, G. Mascia, S. Bombardieri, A. Lucacchini. 2009. Altered amino acid homeostasis in subjects affected by fibromyalgia. *Clin Biochem* 42(10-11):1064-70.

Bazzichi, L., G. Giannaccini, L. Betti, L. Fabbrini, L. Schmid, L. Palego, C. Giacomelli, A. Rossi, L. Giusti, F. De Feo, T. Giuliano, G. Mascia, S. Bombardieri, A. Lucacchini. 2008. ATP, calcium and magnesium levels in platelets of patients with primary fibromyalgia. *Clin Biochem* 41(13):1084-90. Epub 2008 Jul 2.

Bazzichi, L., A. Rossi, G. Massimetti, G. Giannaccini, T. Giuliano, F. De Feo, A. Ciapparelli, L. Dell'Osso, S. Bombardieri. 2007. Cytokine patterns in fibromyalgia and their correlation with clinical manifestations. *Clin Exp Rheumatol.* 25(2):225-30.

Bazzichi, L., A. Rossi, C. Zirafa, F. Monzani, S. Tognini, A. Dardano, F. Santini, M. Tonacchera, M. De Servi, C. Giacomelli, F. De Feo, M. Doveri, G. Massimetti, S. Bombardieri. 2012. Thyroid autoimmunity may represent a predisposition for the development of fibromyalgia? *Rheumatol Int.* 32(2):335-41. doi: 10.1007/s00296-010-1620-1. Epub 2010 Nov 18.

Beckman, J.S., W.H. Koppenol. 1996. Nitric oxide, superoxide, and peroxynitrite: the good, the bad, and ugly. *Am J Physiol.* 271(5 Pt 1):C1424-37.

Bennett, R.M., S.R. Clark, S.M. Campbell, C.S. Burckhardt. 1992. Low levels of somatomedin C in patients with the fibromyalgia syndrome. A possible link between sleep and muscle pain. *Arthritis Rheum.* 35(10):1113-6.

Boomershine, C.S., D. Titova, C. Zhu, A.M. Oeser, M.W. Calcutt, A. Bian, T. Gebretsadik, R. Johnson, C. Michael Stein. 2009. Kynurenine Pathway Activity Linked to Fibromyalgia Fatigue. [Presentation Number: 1991].

Boras, W., J. Lukac, V. Brailo, P. Picek, D. Kordić, I.A. Zilić. 2006. Salivary interleukin-6 and tumor necrosis factor-alpha in patients with recurrent aphthous ulceration. *J Oral Pathol Med* 35(4):241-3.

Boykin Jr., J.V., Baylis, C. 2006. Homocysteine - A Stealth Mediator of Impaired Wound Healing: A Preliminary Study. *Wounds* 18(4):101-116.

Buskila, D, L.R. Odes, L. Neumann, H.S. Odes. 1999. Fibromyalgia in inflammatory bowel disease. *J Rheumatol.* 26(5):1167-71.

Calandre, E.P., J.S. Vilchez, R. Molina-Barea, M. Isabel Tovar, J.M. Garcia-Leiva, J. Hildago, C.M. Rodriquez-Lopez, F. Rico-Villadermoros. 2011. Suicide attempts and risk of suicide in patients with fibromyalgia: a survey in Spanish patients. *Rheumatology* doi:10.1093/rheumatology/ker203First published online: July 12, 2011.

Carwile, J.L., X. Ye, X. Zhou, A.M. Calafat, K.B. Michels. 2011. *J Amer Med Assoc* 306(20):2218-20.

Cedar Sinai. 2013. Retrieved 1/13/2013 online from http://www.cedars-sinai.edu/Patients/Health-Conditions/Adult-Growth-Hormone-Deficiency.aspx.

Chajès, V., A.C.M. Thiébaut, M. Rotival, E. Gauthier, V. Maillard, M.C. Boutron-Ruault, V. Joulin, G.M. Lenoir, F. Clavel-Chapelon. 2008. Serum trans-mono-unsaturated fatty acids are associated with an increased risk of breast cancer in the E3N-EPIC Study. *Am J Epidemiol* 167(11):1312.

Chen, C.L., L.H. Tetri, B.A. Neuschwander-Tetri, S.S. Huang, J.S. Huang. 2011. A mechanism by which dietary trans fats cause atherosclerosis. *J Nutr Biochem* 22(7):649-55.

Ciappuccini, R., T. Ansemant, J.F. Maillefert, C. Tavernier, P. Ornetti. 2010. Aspartame-induced fibromyalgia, an unusual but curable cause of chronic pain. *Clin Exp Rheumatol.* 28(6 Suppl 63):S131-3. Epub 2010 Dec 22.

Cimen, O.B., M.Y. Cimen, Y. Yapici, H. Camdeviren. 2009. Arginase, NOS activities, and clinical features in fibromyalgia patients. *Pain Med.* 10(5):813-8. doi: 10.1111/j.1526-4637.2009.00642.x. Epub 2009 Jun 11.

Challem, Jack and Dolby, Victoria, Homocysteine: The New Cholesterol, Keats Publishing, New Canaan, CT, 1996.

Chavarro, J.E., J.W. Rich-Edwards, B.A. Rosner, W.C. Willett. 2007. Dietary fatty acid intakes and the risk of ovulatory infertility. *Am J Clin Nutr* 85(1):231–7.

Chou, Y.C., M.S. Lee, M.H. Wu, H.L. Shih, T. Yang, C.P. Yu, J.C. Yu, C.A. Sun. 2007. Plasma homocysteine as a metabolic risk factor for breast cancer: findings from a case-control study in Taiwan. *Breast Cancer Res Tr* 101(2):199-205.

Chua, n. H., H.A. Van Suijlekom, K.C. Vissers, L. Arendt-Nielsen, O.H. Wilder-Smith. 2011. Differences in sensory processing between chronic cervical zygapophysial joint pain patients with and without cervicogenic headache. *Cephalalgia*, 31, 953-963.

Chung, K.T., G.S. Gadupudi. 2011. Possible roles of excess tryptophan metabolites in cancer. *Environ Mol Mutagen* 52(2):81-104. doi: 10.1002/em.20588.

Chung, J.H., S.A. Kim, B.Y. Choi, H.S. Lee, S.W. Lee, Y.T. Kim, T.Y. Lee, H.S. Moon. 2012. The association between overactive bladder and fibromyalgia syndrome: A community survey. *Neurourol Urodyn* doi: 10.1002/nau.22277. [Epub ahead of print].

Clarke, G., P. Fitzgerald, J.F. Cryan, E.M. Cassidy, E.M. Quigley, T.G. Dinan. 2009. Tryptophan degradation in irritable bowel syndrome: evidence of indoleamine 2,3-dioxygenase activation in a male cohort. *BMC Gastroenterol.* 9:6. doi: 10.1186/1471-230X-9-6.

Cooke, J.P., D.W. Losordo. 2002. Nitric Oxide and Angiogenesis. *Circulation* (105):2133-5.

Cordero, M.D., M.D. Miguel, I. Carmona-López, P. Bonal, F. Campa, A.M. Moreno-Fernández. 2010. The role of oxidative stress and mitochondrial dysfunction in the pathogenesis of fibromyalgia. *Neuro Endocrinlogy Letters* 31(2):169-173.

Cordero, M.D., M. De Miguel, A.M. Moreno Fernández, I.M. Carmona López, J.G. Maraver, D. Cotán, L.G. Izquierdo, P. Bonal, Francisco Campa, P. Bullon, P. Navas, J.A. Sánchez Alcázar. 2010. Mitochondrial dysfunction and mitophagy activation in blood mononuclear cells of fibromyalgia patients: implications in the pathogenesis of the disease. *Arthritis Res Ther* 12(1): R17. Published online 2010 January 28.

Dantzer, R., J.C. O'Connor, M.A. Lawson, K.W. Kelley. 2011. Inflammation-associated depression: from serotonin to kynurenine. *Psychoneuroendocrinology.* Apr;36(3):426-36. doi: 10.1016/j.psyneuen.2010.09.012. Epub 2010 Oct 30.

Das, I., R.E. Burch, H.K. Hahn. 1984. Effects of zinc deficiency on ethanol metabolism and alcohol and aldehyde dehydrogenase activities. *J Lab Clin Med.* 104(4):610-7.

Dessein, P.H., E. A. Shipton, B.I. Joffe, D.P. Hadebe, A.E. Stanwix, B.A. Van der Merwe. 1999. Hyposecretion of adrenal androgens and the relation of serum adrenal steroids, serotonin and insulin-like growth factor-1 to clinical features in women with fibromyalgia. *Pain* 83(2):313-9.

Dewey, D.L. 1997. *The Facts About Canola Oil. Food For Thought.* Retrieved 6/7/2011 from http://www.dldewey.com/columns/canola.htm

Di Cagno, R., M. De Angelis, S. Auricchio, L. Greco, C. Clarke, M. De Vincenzi, C. Giovannini, M. D'Archivio, F. Landolfo, G. Parrilli, F. Minervini, E. Arendt, M. Gobbetti. 2004. Sourdough bread made from wheat and nontoxic flours and started with selected lactobacilli is tolerated in celiac sprue patients. *Appl Envirion Microbiol.* 70(2):1088-96.

Dickey, W. 2002. Low serum vitamin B12 is common in coeliac disease and is not due to autoimmune gastritis. *Eur J Gastroenterol Hepatol.* Apr;14(4):425-7.

Dixon, S. 2009. Folic Acid and B12 Supplements Increase Cancer Risk. Retrieved 1/11/2013 online from http://coloncancer.about.com/b/2009/11/21/folic-acid-and-b12-supplements-increase-cancer-risk.htm.

Dong, M., Y. Shi, Q. Cheng, M. Hao. 2001. Increased nitric oxide in peritoneal fluid from women with idiopathic infertility and endometriosis. *J Repro Med* 46(10):887-91.

Ebbing, M., K.H. Bønna, O. Nygård, E. Amesen, P.M. Ueland, J.E. Nordrehaug, K. Rasmussen, I. Njolstad, H. Refsum, D.W. Nilsen, A. Tverdal, K. Meyer, S.E. Vollset. 2009. Cancer incidence and mortality after treatment with folic acid and vitamin B12. *J Amer Med Assoc* 18;302(19):2119-26. doi:10.1001/jama.2009.1622.

Edden, R.A., D. Crocetti, H. Zhu, D.L. Gilbert, S.H. Mostofsky. 2012. Reduced GABA concentration in attention-deficit/hyperactivity disorder. *Arch Gen Psychiatry.* Jul;69(7):750-3. doi: 10.1001/archgenpsychiatry.2011.2280.

Edwards, Rob. 2002. Farm salmon is now most contaminated food on shelf; Nationwide. *Sunday Herald,* 20 October 2002. Retrieved 2-20-11 from http://www.robedwards.com/2002/10/farm_salmon_is_.html.

Environmental Working Group. 2012. *Skin Deep Cosmetics Database.* EWG.org. Retrieved 3/14/2012 from http://www.ewg.org/skindeep/.

Epperson, C.N., K. Haga, G.F. Mason, E. Sellers, R. Gueorguieva, W. Zhang, E. Weiss, D.L. Rotham. 2002. Cortical gamma-aminobutyric acid levels across the menstrual cycle in healthy women and those with premenstrual dysphoric disorder: a proton magnetic resonance spectroscopy study. *Arch Gen Psychiatry.* 59(9):851-8.

Fallon, S. 2008. Puffed Grains and Breakfast Cereals, should we eat them? *Nourished Magazine* – Editor's Blog. Retrieved 2/21/2011 from http://editor.nourishedmagazine.com.au/articles/puffedgrains-should-we-eat-them

Finamore, A., M. Massimi, C.L. Devirgiliis, E. Megheri. 2008. Zinc deficiency induces membrane barrier damage and increases neutrophil transmigration in Caco-2 cells. *J Nutr.* 138(9):1664-70.

Fitzgerald, P., E.M. Cassidy, G. Clarke, P. Scully, S. Barry, E.M.M. Quigley, F. Shanahan, J. Cryan, T.G. Dinan. 2008. Tryptophan catabolism in females with irritable bowel syndrome: relationship to interferon-gamma, severity of symptoms and psychiatric co-morbidity. *Neurogastroenterol Motil.* 20(12):1291-7. doi: 10.1111/j.1365-2982.2008.01195.x. Epub 2008 Sep 24.

Flippo, T.S., W.D. Holder Jr. 1993. Neurologic degeneration associated with nitrous oxide anesthesia in patients with vitamin B12 deficiency. *Arch Surg* 128(12):1391-5.

Foerster, B.R., M. Petrou, R.A. Edden, P.C. Sundgren, T. Schmidt-Wilcke, S.E. Lowe, S.E. Harte, D.J. Clauw, R.E. Harris. 2012. Reduced insular γ-aminobutyric acid in fibromyalgia. *Arthritis Rheum*. Feb;64(2):579-83. doi: 10.1002/art.33339.

Food and nutrition board, institute of medicine of the national academies. 2005. *Dietary Reference Intakes for Energy, Carbohydrate, Fiber, Fat, Fatty Acids, Cholesterol, Protein, and Amino Acids(Macronutrients)*. National Academies Press: Washington, D.C.

Fraga, B.P., E.B. Santos, J.P. Farias Neto, J.C. Macieira, L.J. Quitans Jr., A.S. Onofre, J.M. De Satana, P.R. Martins-Filho, L.R. Bonjardim. 2012. Signs and symptoms of temporomandibular dysfunction in fibromyalgic patients. *J Craniofac Surg*. 23(2):615-8. doi: 10.1097/SCS.0b013e31824cd81a.

Fukumura, D., T. Gohongi, A. Kadambi, Y. Izumi, J. Ang, C.O. Yun, D.G. Buerk, P.L. Huang, R.K. Jain. 2001. Predominant role of endothelial nitric oxide synthase in vascular endothelial growth factor induced angiogenesis and vascular permeability. *P Natl Acad Sci USA* 98(5):2604-9.

Gallar, J., C. Morales, V. Freire, M.C. Acosta, C. Belmonte, J.A. Duran. 2009. Decreased corneal sensitivity and tear production in fibromyalgia. *Invest Opthalmol Vis Sci* 50(9):4129-34. doi: 10.1167/iovs.08-3083. Epub 2009 Mar 25.

Geisser, M.E., J.M. Glass, L.D. Rajcevska, D.J. Clauw, D.A. Williams, P.R. Kileny, R.H. Gracely. 2008. Study 1—A Psychophysical Study of Auditory and Pressure Sensitivity in Patients With Fibromyalgia and Healthy Controls. *J Pain*. 9(5);417-22.

Gilman, S., R.D. Chervin, R.A. Koeppe, F.B. Consens, R. Little, H. An, L. Junck, M. Heumann. 2003.Obstructive sleep apnea is related to a thalamic cholinergic deficit in MSA. *Neurology* 61(1):35-9.

Gleason, M.N., R.E. Gosselin, H.C. Hodge. 1957. *Clinical Toxicology of Commercial Products: Acute Poisoning, Home & Farm Edition*. The Williams & Wilkins Co.: Baltimore, M.D.

Goebel, A., S. Buhner, R. Schedel, H. Lochs, G. Sprotte. 2008. Altered intestinal permeability in patients with primary fibromyalgia and in patients with complex regional pain syndrome. *Oxford Journals of Medicine Rheumatology* 47 (8): 1223-1227. doi: 10.1093/rheumatology/ken140.

Greco, L., M. Gobbetti, R. Auricchio, R. Di Mase, F. Landolfo, F. Paparo, R. Di Cagno, M. DeAngelis, C.G. Rizzello, A. Cassone, G. Terrone, L. Timpone, M.

D'Aniello, M. Maglio, R. Troncone, S. Auricchio. 2011. Safety for patients with celiac disease of baked goods made of wheat flour hydrolyzed during food processing. *Clin Gastroenterol Hepatol* 9(1):24-9.

Groth, E. III, 1998. Report. Consumers Union. Retrieved 4/3/11 from http://www.consumersunion.org/food/plasticny698.htm.

Gudin, J. 2004. Expanding Our Understanding of Central Sensitization. Medscape Education. Retrieved from http://www.medscape.org/viewarticle/481798 on February 1, 2013.

Guengerich, F.P. 2008. Cytochrome p450 and chemical toxicology. *Chem Res Toxicol* 21(1):70-83.

Gur, Ali, R. Cevik, K. Nas, L. Colpan, S. Sarac. Cortisol and hypothalamic–pituitary–gonadal axis hormones in follicular-phase women with fibromyalgia and chronic fatigue syndrome and effect of depressive symptoms on these hormones. Published online 2004 March 15. doi: 10.1186/ar1163 PMCID: PMC416440

Halbreich, U., F. Petty, K. Yonkers, G.L. Kramer, A.J. Rush, K.W. Bibi. 1996. Low plasma gamma-aminobutyric acid levels during the late luteal phase of women with premenstrual dysphoric disorder. *Am J Psychiatry* 153(5):718-20.

Harel, Z. and G.S. Tannenbaum. 1993. Dietary protein restriction impairs both spontaneous and growth hormone-releasing factor-stimulated growth hormone release in the rat. *Endocrinology.* 133(3):1035-43.

Harris, C.A., A.F. Miranda, J.J. Tanguay, R.J. Boegman, R.J. Beninger, K. Jhamandas. 1998. Modulation of striatal quinolinate neurotoxicity by elevation of endogenous brain kynurenic acid. *Br J Pharmacol.* 124(2):391-9.

Hedrick, U.P. 1988. A history of horticulture in America to 1860. Portland, Oregon:Timber Press.

Higdon, J. 2003. Coenzyme Q10. Linus Pauling Institute, Oregon State University. Retrieved 12/26/2011 from http://lpi.oregonstate.edu/infocenter/othernuts/coq10/

Himmerich, H., P.A. Beitinger, F. Stephany Fulda, R. Wehrle, J. Linseisen, G. Wolfram, S. Himmerich, K. Gedrich, T.C. Wetter, T. Pollmächer. 2006. Plasma Levels of Tumor Necrosis Factor α and Soluble Tumor Necrosis Factor Receptors in Patients With Narcolepsy. *Arch Intern Med.* 166(16):1739-1743. doi:10.1001/archinte.166.16.1739.

Hörl, W.H. 2008. New Insights Into Intestinal Iron Absorption. *Nephrol. Dial. Transplant.* 23(10):3063-3064.

Hsu, F.C. and S.S. Smith. 2003. Progesterone withdrawal reduces paired-pulse inhibition in rat hippocampus: dependence on GABA(A) receptor alpha4 subunit upregulation. J *Neurophysiol.* 89(1):186-98.

Humira Website. Retrieved 1/11/12 from http://www.humira.com/.

Hyman, M. 2009. Autoimmune Disease: How to stop your body from attacking itself. *Huffpost Living*. Retrieved 4/3/11 from http://www.huffingtonpost.com/dr-mark-hyman/autoimmune-disease-howto_b_283707.html?page=4&show_comment_id=30909196

Isley, W.L., L.E. Underwood, D.R. Clemmons. 1983. Dietary components that regulate serum somatomedin-C concentrations in humans. *J Clin Invest.* 71(2): 175–182. doi: 10.1172/JCI110757 PMCID: PMC436855.

Johnson, C. 2010. Proteins on the Brain: Spinal Tapping for ME/CFS. Phoenix Rising Website. Retrieved 1/11/13 online from http://phoenixrising.me/folder/newsnewsletter/news-2/proteins-on-the-brain-spinal-tapping-for-mecfs-march-2010-by-cort-johnson.

Jones, M., D.C. Kennedy. 1998. *Food and Beverage Sources of Fluoride Exposure*. NoFluoride.com. Retrieved 2/19/2011 from http://www.nofluoride.com/presentations/Fluoride_content_food_%26_beverages.pdf.

Jones, R., K. Franklin, R. Spicer, J. Berry. 1995. Colonic strictures in children with cystic fibrosis on lowstrength pancreatic enzymes. *Lancet* 346:499–500 [letter].

Jones, F. T. (2007). "A Broad View of Arsenic". *Poultry Science* 86(1): 2 –14. PMID 17179408.

Kang, A.H., R.L. Trelstad. 1973. A Collagen Defect in Homocystinuria. *J Clin Invest* 52(10):2571-8.

Keshavarzian, A., S. Choudhary, E.W. Holmes, S. Yong, A. Banan, S. Jakate, J.Z. Fields. Preventing gut leakiness by oats supplementation ameliorates alcohol-induced liver damage in rats. *J Pharmacol Exp Ther.* 299(2):442-8.

Kuchinad, A. P. Schweinhardt, D.A. Seminowicz, P.B. Wood, B.A. Chizh, M.C. Bushnell. 2007. Accelerated brain gray matter loss in fibromyalgia patients: premature aging of the brain? *J Neurosci* 11;27(15):4004-7.

Lachmann, P.J., 2003. Lupus and deoxyribonuclease. *Lupus* 12(3):202-6.

Latimer, E. 2009. Spraying for bugs could increase autoimmune disease risk - Press Release. *American College of Rheumatology*. Retrieved 2/19/11 from https://www.rheumatology.org/about/newsroom/2009/2009_am_18.asp.

Lauria, G., A. Majorana, M. Borgna, R. Lombardi, P. Penza, A. Padovani, P. Sapelli. 2005. Trigeminal small-fiber sensory neuropathy causes burning mouth syndrome. *Pain* 115(3):332-7.

Layer, P., G. Gröger. 1993. Fate of pancreatic enzymes in the human intestinal lumen in health and pancreatic insufficiency. *Digestion*. Suppl 2:10-4.

Lee, L. 2009. *Arthritis.* LitaLee.com Retrieved 2/19/11 from http://www.litalee.com/shopexd.asp?id=132

Levy, Y., J. George, P. Langevitz, D. Harats, R. Doolman, B.A. Sela, Y. Shoenfeld. 1999. Elevated homocysteine levels in patients with Raynaud's syndrome. *J Rheumatol* 26:2383-5.

Liptan, G.L.. 2010. Fascia: A missing link in our understanding of the pathology of fibromyalgia. *J Bodyw Mov Ther.* Jan;14(1):3-12.

Lögters, T.T., M.D. Laryea, M. Jäger, M. Schädel-Höpfner, J. Windolf, S. Flohé, J. Altrichter, M. Scholz, A.N. Paunel-Görgülü. 2010. Kynurenine inhibits chondrocyte proliferation and is increased in synovial fluid of patients with septic arthritis. *J Orthop Res.* 28(11):1490-6. doi: 10.1002/jor.21158.

Lopez-Garcia, E., M.B. Schulze, J.B. Meigs, J.E. Manson, N. Rifai, M.J. Stampfer, W.C. Willett, F. B. Hu. 2005. Consumption of Trans Fatty Acids Is Related to Plasma Biomarkers of Inflammation and Endothelial Dysfunction. *J Nutr* 135(3):562–6.

Lund, N. A. Bengtsson, P. Thorborg. 1986. Muscle tissue oxygen pressure in primary fibromyalgia. *Scand J Rheumatol* 15(2):165-73.

Lupus Foundation of America. 2011. *Living With Lupus: Pain*. Lupus Foundation of America, Inc. Retrieved 6/9/2011 from http://www.lupus.org/webmodules/webarticlesnet/templates/new_ learnliving.aspx?articleid=2255&zoneid=527

Lussana, F., M.L. Zighetti, P. Bucciarelli, M. Cugno, M. Cattaneo. 2003. Blood levels of homocysteine, folate, vitamin B6 and B12 in women using oral contraceptives compared to non-users. *Thromb Res* 112(1-2):37-41.

Maes,M. R. Verkerk, L. Delmeire, A. Van Gastel, F. van Hunsel, S. Scharpé. 2000. Serotonergic markers and lowered plasma branched-chain-amino acid concentrations in fibromyalgia. *Psychiatry Res* Dec 4;97(1):11-20.

Mahfouz, M. 1981. Effect of dietary trans fatty acids on the delta 5, delta 6 and delta 9 desaturases of rat liver microsomes in vivo. *Acta Biol Med Ger* 40(12):1699–1705.

Makris, A., H. Cladd, R.J. Burcombe, J.M. Smith, M. Makris. 2001. Raised Plasma Homocysteine Levels in Women with Metastatic Breast Cancer. *Proc Am Soc Clin Oncol* 20: Abstract 179.

Magaldi, M., L. Moltoni, G. Biasi, R. Marcolongo. 2000. Role of intracellular calcium ions in the physiopathology of fibromyalgia syndrome. *Boll Soc Ital Biol Sper*. 76(1-2):1-4.

Marcus, D.A., C. Bernstein, T.E. Rudy. 2005. Fibromyalgia and headache: an epidemiological study supporting migraine as part of the fibromyalgia syndrome. *Clin Rheumatol* 24(6):595-601. Epub 2005 May 18.

Marcoullis G., Y. Parmentier, J.P. Nicolas, M. Jimenez, P. Gerard. 1980. Cobalamin Malabsorption Due to Nondegradation of R Proteins in the Human Intestine. *J Clin Invest* 66(3):430–40.

Marcus, D.A., C. Bernstein, T.E. Rudy. 2005. Fibromyalgia and headache: an epidemiological study supporting migraine as part of the fibromyalgia syndrome. *Clin Rheumatol* 24(6):595-601. Epub 2005 May 18.

McAlpine, D. and A.R. Palmer. 2002. Blocking GABAergic Inhibition Increases Sensitivity to Sound Motion Cues in the Inferior Colliculus. *The Journal of Neuroscience* 22(4):1443–1453.

McLaren J, A. Prentice, D.S. Charnock-Jones, S.K. Smith. 1996. Vascular endothelial growth factor (VEGF) concentrations are elevated in peritoneal fluid of women with endometriosis. Hum Reprod. 11(1):220-3.

McBeth, J., A.J. Silman, G.J. Macfarlane. 2003. Association of widespread body pain with an increased risk of cancer and reduced cancer survival: a prospective, population-based study. Arthritis Rheum. 48(6):1686-92.

McBride, J. 2000. *B12 deficiency may be more widespread than thought*. USDA Agricultural ResearchService. Retrieved 4/3/11 from http://www.ars.usda.gov/is/pr/2000/000802.htm.

McCormick, J. 2005. A possible link between $24-billion-a-year "antacid" industry and the misery of menopause. *MSNBC News*. Retrieved 4/16/2011 from http://www.msnbc.msn.com/id/40423327/

Melin, .A, P. Sparén , A. Bergqvist. 2007. The risk of cancer and the role of parity among women with endometriosis. *Hum Reprod*. 22(11):3021-6. Epub 2007 Sep 13.

Milla, C.E., C.L. Wielinski, W.J. Warwick. 1994. High-strength pancreatic enzymes. *Lancet*;343:599 [letter].

Molecular Psychiatry 2004 Volume 9, advance online publication doi:10.1038/sj.mp.4001476. Retrieved online 1/09/2013 from http://www.eurekalert.org/pub_releases/2004-02/mp-alb020204.php.

Molloy, A.M., P.N. Kirke, J.F. Troendle, H. Burke, M. Sutton, L.C. Sutton, L.C. Brody, J.M. Scott, J.L. Mills. 2009. Maternal Vitamin B12 Status and Risk of Neural Tube Defects in a Population With High Neural Tube Defect Prevalence and No Folic Acid Fortification. *Pediatrics* Vol. 123 No. 3, pp. 917-923 (doi: 10.1542/peds.2008-1173) Article.

Morris, M.C., D.A. Evans, J.L. Bienias, C.C. Tangney, D.A. Bennett, N. Aggarwal, J. Schneider, R.S. Wilson. 2003. Dietary fats and the risk of incident Alzheimer disease. *Arch Neurol* 60(2):194–200.

Moschiano. F., D. D'Amico, S. Usai, L. Grazzi, M. Di Stefano, E. Ciusani, N. Erba, G. Bussone. 2008. Homocysteine plasma levels in patients with migraine with aura. *Neurol Sci* 29(Suppl. 1):S173-5.163. MSNBC. 2011. Having a baby makes mom's body turn on itself. *MSNBC News*. Retrieved 6/7/2011

Myhill, S. 2007. Lack of stomach acid-hypochlorhydria-can cause lots of problems. *ProHealth*. Retrieved 4/25/2011 from http://www.prohealth.com/library/showarticle.cfm?libid=13388

Nacir, B., H. Genc, B. Duvur Cakit, A. Karagoz, H.R. Erdem. 2012. Evaluation of upper extremity nerve conduction velocities and the relationship between fibromyalgia and carpaltunnel syndrome. *Arch Med Res.* doi: 10.1016/j.arcmed.2012.07.004. Epub 2012 Jul 25.

Nakamura, Y., H. Yasuoka, M. Tsuijmoto, K. Yoshidome, M. Nakamura, K. Kakudo. 2006a. Nitric oxide in breast cancer: induction of vascular endothelial growth factor-C and correlation with metastasis and poor prognosis. *Clin Cancer Res* 12(4):1201-7.

National Cancer Institute. 2005. Understanding Cancer Series. Retreived 1/11/13 online from http://www.cancer.gov/cancertopics/understandingcancer/angiogenesis/page1.

National Institutes of Health. 2009. *Dietary Supplement Fact Sheet: Magnesium.* U.S. Department of Health and Human Services. Retrieved 5/9/2011 from http://ods.od.nih.gov/factsheets/magnesium/.

National Institutes of Health. 2010. *Vitamin B12*. U.S. Department of Health and Human Services. Retrieved 4/3/11 from http://ods.od.nih.gov/factsheets/vitaminb12/

National Institutes of Health. 2002. *Women with Endometriosis have Higher Rates of Some Diseases.* U.S. Department of Health and Human Services. Retrieved 3/4/2012 from http://www.nih.gov/news/pr/sep2002/nichd-26.htm.

National Institutes of Health. 2011. Office of Dietary Supplements. Retrieved 1/9/2013 online from http://ods.od.nih.gov/factsheets/Zinc-HealthProfessional/

Nickel, J.C., D.A. Tripp, M. Pontari, R. Moldwin, R. Mayer, L.K. Carr, R. Doggweiler, C.C. Yang, N. Mishra, J. Nordling. 2010. Interstitial cystitis/painful bladder syndrome and associated medical conditions with an emphasis on irritable bowel syndrome, fibromyalgia and chronic fatigue syndrome. *J Urol.* 184(4):1358-63. doi: 10.1016/j.juro.2010.06.005. Epub 2010 Aug 17.

Nordeman, L., R. Gunnarsson, K. Mannerkorpi. 2012. Prevalence and characteristics of widespread pain in female primary health care patients with chronic low back pain. *Clin J Pain* 28:65-72. doi: 10.1097/AJP.0b013e318223622c.

Northwestern University (2001, June 26). Chemists Characterize Regulators of Zinc Intake And Export in Cells. *ScienceDaily.*

Nöthlings, U., L.R. Wilkens, S.P. Murhpy, J.H. Hankin, B.E. Henderson, L.N. Kolonel. Meat and Fat Intake as Risk Factors for Pancreatic Cancer: The Multiethnic Cohort Study. *J Natl Cancer Ins* 97(19):1458.

Olsson, S.K., M. Samuelsson, P. Saetre, L. Lindström, E.G. Jönsson, C. Nordin, G. Engberg, S. Erhardt, M. Landén. 2010. Elevated Levels of Kynurenic Acid in the Cerebrospinal Fluid of Patients with Bipolar Disorder. *J Psychiatry Neurosci* 35(3):195-9.

O'Neill, S., C. Manniche, T. Graven-Nielsen, L. Arendt-Nielsen. 2007. Generalized deep-tissue hyperalgesia in patients with chronic low-back pain. *European Journal of Pain,* 11, 415-420.

Ortancil, O. A. Sanli, R. Eryuksel, A. Basaran, H. Ankarali. 2010. Association between serum ferritin level and fibromyalgia syndrome. *Eur J Clin Nutr.* Mar;64(3):308-12. doi: 10.1038/ejcn.2009.149. Epub 2010 Jan 20.

Oxford Journals Press. *Hum. Reprod.* Update (2007) 13 (3): 225-238. doi: 10.1093/humupd/dml063 First published online: February 16, 2007. Retrieved 1/11/13 online from http://humupd.oxfordjournals.org/content/13/3/225.abstract?ijkey=6120eec69b9549806 7ce0077e1b7e461933f33f4&keytype2=tf_ipsecsha.

Panerai, A.E., J. Vecchiet, P. Panzeri, P. Meroni, S. Scarone, E. Pizzigallo, M.A. Giamberardino, P. Sacerdote. 2002. Peripheral blood mononuclear cell beta-endorphin concentration is decreased in chronic fatigue syndrome and fibromyalgia but not in depression: preliminary report. *Clin J Pain.* 18(4):270-3.

Park, J.H., P. Phothimat, C.T. Oates, M. Hernanz-Schulman, N.J. Olsen. 1998. Use of P-31 magnetic resonance spectroscopy to detect metabolic abnormalities in muscles of patients with fibromyalgia. *Arthritis Rheum* 41(3):406-13.

Pellegrino, M.J., D. Van Fossen, C. Gordon, J.M. Ryan, G.W. Waylonis. 1989. Prevalence of mitral valve prolapse in primary fibromyalgia: a pilot investigation. *Arch Phys Med Rehabil* 70(7):541-3.

Peres, M.F., E. Zukerman, C.A. Senne Soares, E.O. Alonso, B.F. Santos, M.H. Faulhaber. 2004. Cerebrospinal fluid glutamate levels in chronic migraine. *Cephalalgia* 24(9):735-9.

Pham, C.T.N. 2008. Neutrophil Serine Proteases Fine-Tune the Inflammatory Response. *Int J Biochem Cell Biol.* 40(6-7):1317-1333.

Phelps, J.E. 2005. *Chronic Fatigue, Fluoride & Heavy Metals.* Elektralife.com. Retrieved 2/18/2011 from http://elektralife.com/index.php?option=com_content&view=article&id=85&Itemid=92.

Pimental, M., D. Wallace, D. Hallegua, E. Chow, Y. Kong, S. Park, H.C. Lin. 2004. A link between irritable bowel syndrome and fibromyalgia may be related to findings on lactulose breath testing. *Ann Rheum Dis* 63:450-452 doi:10.1136/ard.2003.011502

Pinelli, A., S. Govoni, C. Ossi, F. Battaini, B.R. Caimi, S. Trivulzio. 1985. Kynurenine may directly interact with GABA receptors in rat brain. *Pharmacology* 30(5):255-8.

Pitcher, D., R. Grahame. 1982. Mitral valve prolapse and joint hypermobility: evidence for a systemic connective tissue abnormality? *Ann Rheum Dis* 41(4):352-4.

Plengvidhya, V., F. Breidt Jr., Z. Lu, H.P. Fleming. 2007. DNA fingerprinting of lactic acid bacteria in sauerkraut fermentations. *Appl Environ Mircrobiol* 73(23):7697-702.

Plioplys, A.V., S. Plioplys. 1997. Amantadine and L-Carnitine Treatment of Chronic Fatigue Syndrome. *Neuropsychobiology* 35(1):16-23.

Powell C.J. 1999. Colonic toxicity from pancreatins: a contemporary safety issue. *Lancet* Mar 13;353(9156):911-5.

Powell, C.J. 1999. Pancreatic enzymes and fibrosing colonopathy. *Lancet* 354:251 [letter].

Quinzii, C.M., M. Hirano. 2010. Coenzyme Q and mitochondrial disease. 2010. *Dev Disabil Res Rev.* 16(2):183-8. doi: 10.1002/ddrr.108.

Raloff, J. 1989. Dioxin: Paper's Trace. *Science News* 135(7):104.

Reed Business Information Ltd. 2006. Six years of fast-food supersizes monkeys. *NewScientist* (2556):21. Retrieved 5/24/2011 from http://www.newscientist.com/article/mg19025565.000-sixyears-of-fastfood-fats-supersizes-monkeys.html.

Regland, B., M. Andersson, L. Abrahamsson, J. Bagby, L.E. Dyrehag, C.G. Gottfries. 1997. Increased concentrations of homocysteine in the cerebrospinal fluid in patients with fibromyalgia and chronic fatigue syndrome. *Scand J Rheumatol* 26(4):301-7.

Reuter, S.E., A.M. Evans. 2010. Long-chain Acylcarnitine Deficiency in Patients with Chronic Fatigue Syndrome. Potential Involvement of Altered Carnitine Palmitoyltransferase-I Activity. *Journal of Internal Medicine*:1365-2796.

Reuter, S., A. Heinz, M. Sieren, R. Wiewrodt, E.W. Gelfand, M. Stassen, R. Buhl, C. Taube. 2008. Mast cell-derived tumor necrosis factor is essential for allergic airway disease. *Eur Respir J.* 31(4):773-82. Epub 2007 Dec 19.

Reyero, F., G. Ponce, R. Rodriguez-Jimenez, P. Fernandez-Dapica, D. Taboada, V. Martin, M. Navio, M.A. Jimenez-Arriero, J. Hoenicka, T. Palomo. 2011. High frequency of childhood ADHD history in women with fibromyalgia. *Eur Psychiatry.* Nov; 26(8):482-3. doi: 10.1016/j.eurpsy.2010.03.012. Epub 2010 Jul 10.

Riedel, W., H. Layka, G. Neeck. 1998. Secretory pattern of GH, TSH, thyroid hormones, ACTH, cortisol, FSH, and LH in patients with fibromyalgia syndrome following systemic injection of the relevant hypothalamic-releasing hormones. *Z Rheumatol* 57 Suppl 2:81-7.

Roan, S. 2011. Trans fats and saturated fats could contribute to depression. *Sydney Morning Herald.* Retrieved 5/23/2011 from http://www.smh.com.au/lifestyle/wellbeing/food-with-bad-fats-linked-todepression-study-finds-20110127-1a6vy.html

Romano, T.J., J.W. Stiller. 1994. Magnesium Deficiency in Fibromyalgia Syndrome. *Journal of Nutritional and Environmental Medicine.* Vol. 4, No. 2, pages 165-167.

Rubio-Diaz, D.E., M.E. Pozza, J. Dimitrakov, J.P. Gilleran, M.M. Giusti, J.L. Stella, L.E. Rodriguez-Saona, C.A. Buffington. 2009. A candidate serum biomarker for bladder pain syndrome/interstitial cystitis. *Analyst* 134(6):1133-7. doi: 10.1039/b901736d. Epub 2009 Apr 16.

Samborski, W., J.K. Lacki, K.E. Wiktorowicz. 1996. The lymphocyte phenotype in patients with primary fibromyalgia. *Ups J Med Sci.* 101(3):251-6.

Schutzer, S.E., T.E. Angel, T. Liu, A.A. Schepmoes, T.R. Clauss, J.N. Adkins, D.G. Camp, B.K. Holland, J. Berquist, P.K. Coyle, R.D. Smith, B.A. Fallon, B.H. Natelson. 2011. Distinct cerebrospinal fluid proteomes differentiate post-treatment lyme disease from chronic fatigue syndrome. *PLoS One* 6(2):e17287. doi: 10.1371/journal.pone.0017287.

Sendur, O.F., E. Tastaban, Y. Turan, C. Ulman. 2008. The relationship between serum trace element levels and clinical parameters in patients with fibromyalgia. *Rheumatol Int.* 28(11):1117-21. doi: 10.1007/s00296-008-0593-9. Epub 2008 May 22.

Sendur, O.F., Y. Turan, E. Tastaban, C. Yenisey, M. Serter. 2009. Serum antioxidants and nitric oxide levels in fibromyalgia: a controlled study. *Rheumatol Int.* 29(6):629-33. Epub 2008 Oct 14.

Sieverling, C. 2002. Paul Cheney, M.D., on SSRIs and stimulants for chronic fatigue syndrome: frying the brain? *ProHealth*: June 5, 2002. Retrieved 4/25/2011 from http://www.prohealth.com/library/showarticle.cfm?libid=8480

Silver, R.M., M.P. Heyes, J.C. Maize, B. Quearry, M. Vionnet-Fuasset. 1990. Scleroderma, Fasciitis, and Eosinophilia Associated with the Ingestion of Tryptophan. *N Engl J Med* 322:874-881 March 29, 1990 DOI: 10.1056/NEJM199003293221302.

Shah, M.A., S. Feinberg, E. Krishnan. 2006. Sleep-disordered breathing among women with fibromyalgia syndrome. *J Clin Rheumatol.* 2006 12(6):277-81.

Slotkoff, A. T., D. A. Radulovic, D. J. Clauw. 1997. The Relationship between Fibromyalgia and the Multiple Chemical Sensitivity Syndrome. *Annals of Internal Medicine* Vol. 26, No. 5 , Pages 364-367.

Solano, C., A. Martinez, L. Becerril, A. Vargas, J. Figueroa, C. Navarro, C. Ramos-Remus, M. Martinez-Lavin. 2009. Autonomic dysfunction in fibromyalgia assessed by the Composite Autonomic Symptoms Scale (COMPASS). *J Clin Rheumatol* 15(4):172-6. doi: 10.1097/RHU.0b013e3181a1083d.

Spitzer, A.R., M. Broadman. 2010. Treatment of the narcoleptiform sleep disorder in chronic fatigue syndrome and fibromyalgia with sodium oxybate. *Pain Pract*. 10(1):54-9. doi: 10.1111/j.1533-2500.2009.00334.x.

Sprott, H. A. Müller, H. Heine. 1998. Collagen cross-links in fibromyalgia syndrome. *Z Rheumatol.* 57 Suppl 2:52-5.

Staud, R. 2008. Autonomic dysfunction in fibromyalgia syndrome: postural orthostatic tachycardia. *Curr Rheumatol Rep* 10(6):463-6.

Stitt, P., M. Knickelbine, S. Knickelbine. 1980. *Fighting the food giants*. Natural Press: Manitowoc, WI.

Sublette, M.E., H.C. Galfalyy, D. Fuchs, M. Lapidus, M.F. Grunebaum, M.A. Oquendo, J.J. Mann, T.T. Postolache. 2011. Plasma kynurenine levels are elevated in suicide attempters with major depressive disorder. *Brain Behav Immun.* 25(6):1272-8. doi: 10.1016/j.bbi.2011.05.002. Epub 2011 May 14.

Swezey, R.L., J. Adams. 1999. Fibromyalgia: A Risk Factor for Osteoporosis. *J Rheumatol* 26(12):2642-4.

Sy, Ng. 1999. Hair calcium and magnesium levels in patients with fibromyalgia: a case center study. *J Manipulative Physiol Ther.* 22(9):586-93.

Tavares, R.G., C.I. Tasca, C.E. Santos, L.B. Alves, L.O. Porciúncula, T. Emanuelli, D.O. Souza. 2002. Quinolinic acid stimulates synaptosomal glutamate release and inhibits glutamate uptake into astrocytes. *Neurochem Int.* 40(7):621-7.

Taylor, D.A. 2004. Funky Chicken: Consumes Exposed to Arsenic in Poultry. *Environ Health Persp* 112(1):A50.

Tipton, K.D., 2001. Gender differences in protein metabolism. *Curr Opin Clin Nutr Metab Care.* 4(6):493-8.

Torresani, C., S. Bellafiore, G. De Panfilis. 2009. Chronic urticaria is usually associated with fibromyalgia syndrome. *Acta Derm Venereol.* 89(4):389-92. doi: 10.2340/00015555-0653.

Untersmayr, .E, E. Jensen-Jarolim. 2006. The effect of gastric digestion on food allergy. *Curr Opin Allergy Clin Immunol* 6:214-219.

Untersmayr E, Bakos N, Scholl I, et al. 2005. Anti-ulcer drugs promote IgE formation toward dietary antigens in adult patients. *FASEB J* 19:656-658.

Uratsune, K., H., K. Yamaguti, M. Takahashi, et al. 1994. Acylcarnitine Deficiency in Chronic Fatigue Syndrome. *Clinical Infectious Disease* 18(3 Supplement 1): S62-S67.

U.S. Dept of Health and Human Services. 2003. *Trans Fat Press Conference.* U.S. Food and Drug Administration. Retrieved 5/24/2011 from http://www.hhs.gov/news/speech/2003/030709.html.

U.S. Dept of Health and Human Services. 2011. *How to Understand and Use the Nutrition Facts Label.* U.S. Food and Drug Administration. Retrieved 5/23/2011 from http://www.fda.gov/food/labelingnutrition/consumerinformation/ucm078889.htm

Vaerøy, H, R. Helle, O. Førre, E. Kåss, L. Terenius. 2000. Elevated CSF levels of substance P and high incidence of Raynaud phenomenon in patients with fibromyalgia: new features for diagnosis. *Boll Soc Ital Biol Sper.* 76(1-2):1-4.

van Staa, T.P., P. Geusens, J.W. Bijlsma, H.G. Leufkens, C. Cooper. 2006. Clinical assessment of the long-term risk of fracture in patients with rheumatoid arthritis. *Arthritis Rheum* 54(10):3104-12.

Veale, D., G. Kavanagh, J.F. Fielding, O. Fitzgerald. 1991. Primary fibromyalgia and the irritable bowel syndrome: different expressions of a common pathogenetic process. *Br J Rheumatol.* 30(3):220-2.

Viola-Saltzman, M. N.F. Watson, A. Bogart, J. Goldberg, D. Buchwald. 2010. High prevalence of restless legs syndrome among patients with fibromyalgia: a controlled cross-sectional study. *Journal of Clinical Sleep Medicine* vol 6: pp 423-427.

Wei, X.H.; Zang, Y., Wu, C.Y., Xu, J.T., Xin, W.J., and Liu, X.G. (2007). "Perisciatic administration of recombinant rat TNF-alpha induces mechanical allodynia via upregulation of TNF-alpha in dorsal root ganglia and in spinal dorsal horn: The role of NF-kappa B pathway". *Experimental Neurology* 205: 471-484.

Weinberg, E.D. 1996. The role of iron in cancer. *Eur J Cancer Prev*. 5(1):19-36.

Wenyan, Li., T. Zheng, J. Wang, B.T. Altura, B.M. Altura. 1999. Extracellular magnesium regulates effects of vitamin B6, B12 and folate on homocysteinemia-induced depletion of intracellular free magnesium ions in canine cerebral vascular smooth muscle cells: possible relationship to [Ca2+]i, atherogenesis and stroke. *Neurosci Lett.* 19 274 (2):83-6 10553943.

Wikner, J., U. Hirsch, L. Wetterberg, S. Röjdmark. 1998. Fibromyalgia--a syndrome associated with decreased nocturnal melatonin secretion. *Clin Endocrinol (Oxf)* 49(2):179-83.

Wilson, L.H., Eliason, M.J., Leiferman, K.M., Hull, C.M., Powell, D.L. 2011. Treatment of refractory chronic urticaria with tumor necrosis factor–alfa inhibitors. *Journal of the American Academy of Dermatology* Volume 64, Issue 6 , Pages 1221-1222.

Wingenfeld, K., C. Heim, I. Schmidt, D. Wagner, G. Meinlschmidt, D.H. Hellhammer. 2007. HPA Axis Reactivity and Lymphocyte Glucocorticoid Sensitivity in Fibromyalgia Syndrome and Chronic Pelvic Pain. *Psychosom Med* January 2008 vol. 70 no. Published online before print December 24, 2007, doi:10.1097/PSY.0b013e31815ff3ce.

Wolfe, F., I.J. Russell, G. Vipraio, K. Ross, J. Anderson. 1997. Serotonin levels, pain threshold, and fibromyalgia symptoms in the general population. *J Rheumatol* Mar;24(3):555-9.

Wood, P.B., J.C. Patterson 2nd, J.J. Sunderland, K.H. Tainter, M.F. Glabus, D.L. Lilien. 2007. Reduced presynaptic dopamine activity in fibromyalgia syndrome demonstrated with positron emission tomography: a pilot study. *J Pain* 8(1):51-8. Epub 2006 Oct 4.

Wood, P.B., M.F. Glabus, R. Simpson, J.C. Patterson 2nd. 2009. Changes in gray matter density in fibromyalgia: correlation with dopamine metabolism. *J Pain.* 10(6):609-18. Epub 2009 Apr 23.

Wu, M.Y., K.H. Chao, J.H. Yang, T.H. Lee, Y.S. Yang, H.N. Ho. 2003. Nitric oxide synthesis is increased in the endometrial tissue of women with endometriosis. *Hum Reprod* 18(12):2688-94.

Yasutomo, K., T. Horiuchi, S. Kagami, H. Tsukamoto, C. Hashimura, M. Urushihara, Y. Kuroda. 2001. Mutation of DNASE1 in people with systemic lupus erythematosus. *Nat Genet* 28(4):313-4.

Yeh, Yu-Yan; Yeh, Shaw-mei. "Homocysteine-Lowering Action Is Another Potential Cardiovascular Protective Factor of Aged Garlic Extract1-3." *The Journal of Nutrition.* American Society for Nutritional Sciences. 2006. HighBeam Research. 25 Jan. 2013.

Yeh GY, Davis RB, Phillips RS. Use of Complementary Therapies in Patients With Cardiovascular Disease *The American Journal of Cardiology* 2006; 98(5): 673-680.

Yiamouyiannis, J. 1986. *Fluoride: The Aging Factor*. Health Action Press: Deleware, OH.

Yunus M.B., J.W. Dailey, J.C. Aldag, A.T. Masi, P.C. Jobe. 1992. Plasma tryptophan and other amino acids in primary fibromyalgia: a controlled study. *J Rheumatol.* Jan;19(1):90-4.

Zasshi, Shokuhin Eiseigaku. Fukuwatari T, Toriochi M, Ohta M, Sasaki R, Shibata K. 2004. Metabolic disturbance of tryptophan-nicotinamide conversion pathway by putative endocrine disruptors, bisphenol A and styrene monomer. Shokuhin Eiseigaku Zasshi. *Journal of the Food Hygienic Society of Japan* [2004, 45(1):1-7].

Zhan, S., G.Q. Cai, A. Zheng, Y. Wang, J. Jia, H. Fang, Y. Yang, M. Hu, Q. Ding. 2011. Tumor necrosis factor-alpha regulates the Hypocretin system via mRNA degradation and ubiquitination. *Biochim Biophys Acta.* 1812(4):565-71. doi: 10.1016/j.bbadis.2010.11.003. Epub 2010 Nov 18.

Zhang, F., Y.L. Siow, O. K. 2004. Hyperhomcysteinemia activates NF-kappaB and inducible nitric oxide synthase in the kidney. *Kidney Int.* 65(4):1327-38.